EASY RUNNING PLANS

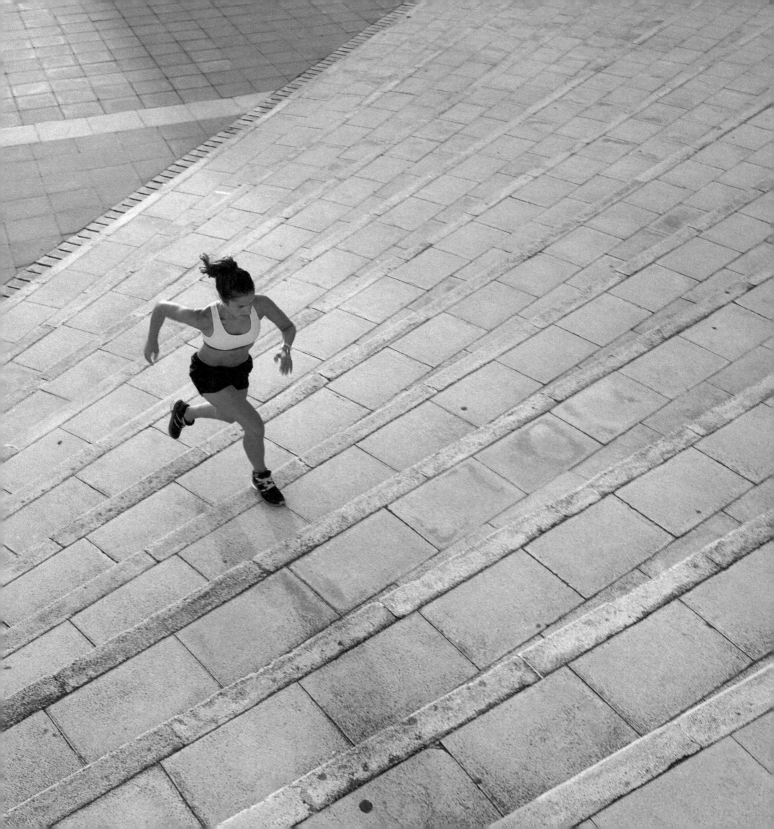

EASY RUNNING PLANS

Total-Body Training for Speed, Strength, and Endurance

Jeff Gaudette

ROCKRIDGE
PRESS

For general information on our other products and services or to obtain technical support, please contact our Customer Care Department within the United States at (866) 744-2665, or outside the United States at (510) 253-0500.

Rockridge Press publishes its books in a variety of electronic and print formats. Some content that appears in print may not be available in electronic books, and vice versa.

TRADEMARKS: Rockridge Press and the Rockridge Press logo are trademarks or registered trademarks of Callisto Media Inc. and/or its affiliates, in the United States and other countries, and may not be used without written permission. All other trademarks are the property of their respective owners. Rockridge Press is not associated with any product or vendor mentioned in this book.

Interior and Cover Designer: Sean Doyle
Art Producer: Michael Hardgrove
Editor: Sam Eichner
Illustration © Christian Papazoglakis, 2019.
Photography © Stocksy/Guille Faingold, p. ii; iStock/lzf, pp. xi, 28; iStock/Irina Vodneva, p. 2; Shutterstock/Dean Drobot, p. 7; iStock/mapodile, p. 8; iStock/Pekic, p. 13; iStock/Jelena Hinic, p. 16; iStock/Dusan Petkovic, p. 27; Shutterstock/kikovic, p. 39; Stocksy/Jovo Jovanovic, p. 40; iStock/Karel Noppe, p. 59; Creative Market/New York Art Store, p. 62; Shutterstock/Dirima, p. 76; iStock/FatCamera, p. 101; iStock/baona, p. 102; iStock/PeopleImages, p. 110.

ISBN: Print 978-1-64611-200-5 | eBook 978-1-64611-201-2
R0

I'd like to dedicate this book to my family,
Karen, Javrila, Luis, Emiliano, and Ethan.

TABLE OF CONTENTS

INTRODUCTION: DEVELOPING YOUR TOTAL-BODY RUNNING PLAN

My name is Jeff Gaudette, and I have been an avid runner for 20 years. I started my running career as a competitive athlete, earning numerous All-American awards while attending Brown University. After college, I competed professionally, racing across the globe and recording Olympic-qualifying marks in the 10,000 meters and marathon.

My competitive running career afforded me the opportunity to train under some of the best coaches in the world. Learning the science behind training and how it translated to helping others inspired me to begin coaching in 2005. Since that time, I've coached thousands of runners, written extensively for some of the largest running publications, and presented my coaching philosophy at prestigious coaching conferences.

I list these accomplishments not to toot my own horn, but to help you understand why I wanted to write this book. As an athlete, I made all the same mistakes most new runners make. I tried to run too hard every day, I didn't give my body the recovery time it needed, and I didn't realize the importance of strength work and stretching. My idea of training was just running as many miles as I could.

Unfortunately, this mind-set forced me to retire from competitive running after career-ending injuries. I missed numerous races due to injuries, and trivializing strength work and stretching hampered my performance and potential. I look back on these days and wish I could impart to my younger self the knowledge I've gained in my 13 years as a coach. Although I can't change my past, I can help you avoid those same mistakes.

My hope is that after reading this book you will understand the value of a total-body running plan. You'll understand why posture and running form are integral to your performance, and how to properly improve these elements. You'll understand the effectiveness of strength training to prevent injuries and improve performance. And you'll understand how to structure your workouts to get the most out of your runs.

For the past few years, my passion has been translating highly technical scientific research and real-life data from runners I've coached into approachable, actionable advice for runners like you. Featuring easy-to-follow, highly effective training regimens, this book is a culmination of my years of learning as an athlete, coach, and lover of science. I'm excited to share my knowledge with you and help you become the best runner you can be.

Why This Book

Running is simple, right? Lace up your shoes, get out the door, put one foot in front of the other, and try to run more each day.

The unfortunate truth is that becoming a better runner while staying healthy involves a lot more than just logging mileage. Supplemental drills, stretches, strength exercises, and running-specific workouts are essential to improving your overall running performance. I can virtually guarantee that runners who ignore these training elements will eventually get injured or hit a wall in their personal progress.

Some running books may include these crucial elements, but their fitness plans can be impractical and difficult to follow. Many running books list exercises but leave it to the reader to figure out how to incorporate them. These books can also be overly technical, operating under the assumption that you have a PhD in exercise physiology.

This book takes a different approach to your total-body running plan.

1. It's structured to be as easy to use as possible. Everything I cover in this book can (and will) be incorporated into your training regimen. There's no guesswork.

2. I include only the most effective stretches, drills, and strength exercises. Plus, the routines require minimal to no equipment and can be performed at home.

3. This book is designed to be useful for runners at every skill level. It will help both new and experienced runners understand why a total-body approach to running actually works.

Choose Your Own Path

This book is broken into four parts, each designed to help guide you through the process of becoming a better runner.

Before You Lace Up (chapters 1 and 2)
This section helps you get motivated and ensures you have all the right equipment to get started. If you need help setting goals, finding the right shoes, or dressing for weather conditions, this section is the best place to look.

The Fundamentals (chapters 3 to 5)
These chapters take a deep dive into running posture, building a strong running stride, and helping you stay injury-free. This section covers why proper form is important and how to improve it.

Putting in the Work (chapters 6 to 8)
In these three chapters, I detail specific technique drills, strength workouts, and types of runs to help you become a total-body runner. I also explain the science behind these workouts and discuss how to include them in your plan.

Time to Train (chapter 9)
This chapter contains sample training plans that tie together the information and routines discussed in the other chapters. There are training schedules for different skill levels: New Runners (see page 113), Noncompetitive Novices (see page 118), and Noncompetitive Intermediate Runners (see page 122). I've also included training schedules for different goals: Running Your First 5k (see page 126), Running Your First 10k (see page 132), Running Your First Half Marathon (see page 138), and Running Your First Marathon (see page 144). If you're looking for a plan to start following right away, you can jump to the appropriate page and work backward from there.

Developing Your Total-Body Running Plan

Although chapter 9 contains a variety of training plans, I realize that not every plan will work for every type of runner. Perhaps you want to run fewer days per week, or you'd rather do your strength work in the gym or your long runs on Saturday. These scenarios are perfectly reasonable, which is why I provide the science behind the drills, workouts, and runs in chapters 6 through 8.

If you're going to develop your own plan, though, here are some important components to keep in mind:

- Strength training (see chapter 7) is vital to staying healthy and improving performance. You should have at least three days of strength training each week.

- Finding and maintaining your ideal stride is essential. You can do the stretching routine in chapter 4 and the technique drills in chapter 6 each week to ensure you're running with good form.

- A running or strength workout is only beneficial if you're able to properly recover and absorb the benefits. In chapter 5, I discuss how to recover between workouts, and even give you a simple routine to follow. Don't skimp on recovery.

- The easiest way to deal with running injuries is to prevent them from occurring. Include the injury-prevention work from chapter 5 in your plan and always stop to treat injuries as soon as you notice them.

- Include a variety of runs in your training schedule. Simply running hard every day will quickly lead to plateaus. Use the various runs in chapter 8 to mix up your training.

- Stay on the recommended pace for the runs provided in chapter 8 to get the most out of every workout. Most importantly, do not run too fast on your easy days. Running faster on easy days does not help you improve, but leads to injuries and causes you to plateau.

Rules of the Road

If you're building your own running plan, here are some hard-and-fast rules you should follow to make sure you stay healthy and continue to make progress.

1. **Do not perform harder or faster running workouts on back-to-back days.** You should have at least one day of rest or one day of easy running between every workout.

2. **Always perform your strength training after your run.** Doing so guarantees you're not too tired to run. And keep in mind: These workouts don't have to be performed immediately after you run. They can be done later in the day—just don't do them before your run.

3. **Don't increase your mileage by more than 40 percent in one week.** For example: If you ran a total of 15 miles the previous week, the maximum you should run the next week is 21.

4. **Include at least three of the suggested strength training routines in your weekly schedule.** Don't repeat the same strength training three or four times per week just because you like it.

5. **For strength workouts, follow the motto, "Hard days hard, easy days easy."** This rule means harder strength workouts, such as leg day and plyometrics, should be performed on the same day as your harder or faster runs, while easier strength workouts, such as core and hip routines, should be performed on easy or rest days. Following this method will improve your recovery time.

Before You Run

- Whenever I introduce a new stretching, technique, or strength routine in the book, I also provide a short abbreviation in parentheses. (For example, the abbreviation for the Core Routine in chapter 8 is CR.)

- In chapter 9, these codes are included in the sample training schedules, complete with corresponding page numbers.

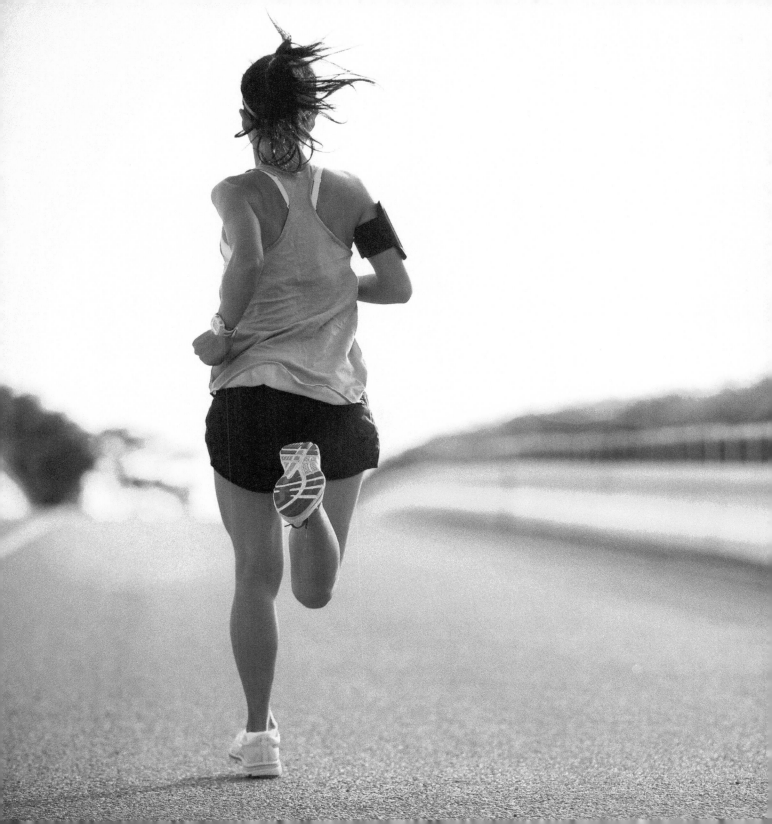

PART ONE

BEFORE YOU LACE UP

Before you get started with your running and strength workouts, it's important you have the right mind-set and motivations. You'll also need the correct clothing, shoes, and equipment. In these first two chapters, I'll make sure you have everything you need to hit the ground running (pun intended).

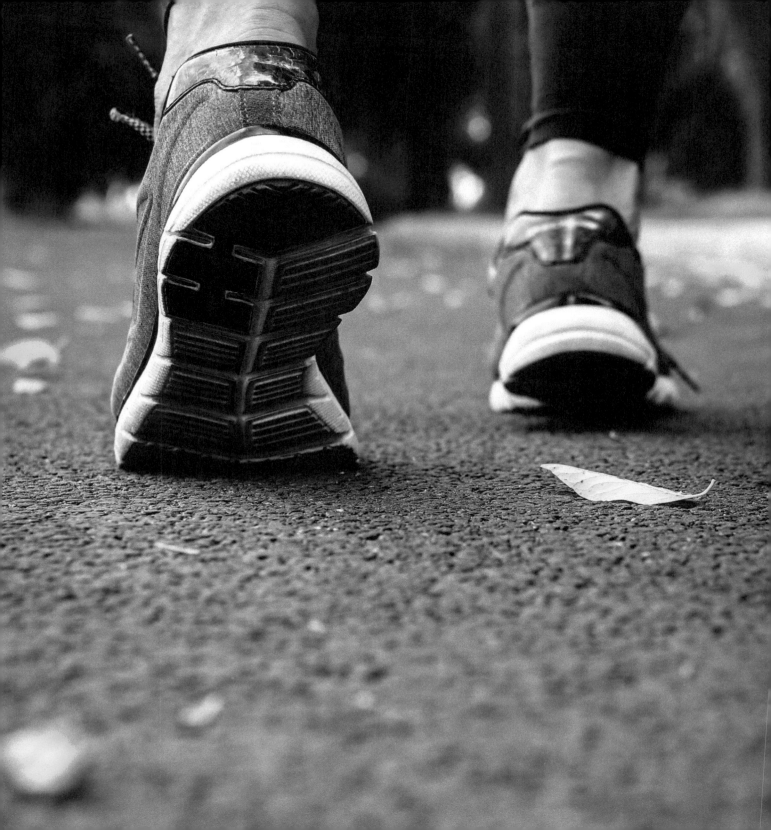

CHAPTER ONE

Running: What Is It Good For?

Fail to plan, plan to fail—this statement is as true for running as it is for any sport or life endeavor. You can't create a road map if you don't know where you want to end up, so the first step is to identify and set a goal. Your goal can be something specific, like finishing a marathon or running your first 5k. Or you can focus on something more abstract, such as improving your overall fitness or staying injury-free. In this chapter, I'll help you uncover what you hope to accomplish as you begin your running journey.

Find Your Drive

"Why do you run?"

Ask a dozen runners this question, and you might get a dozen different answers. Typically, runners run to:

- Relieve stress
- Improve heart conditioning
- Lose weight
- Become a better overall athlete
- Train for a specific race
- Stay (or at least feel) young
- Meditate
- Improve blood pressure
- Increase overall energy
- Make new friends and have fun

You probably have several motivations, some of which may not be on that list. It's important to find your motivation and keep it in mind because, at some point, training will become difficult. You'll get busy, you'll be tired after a long day, you'll be sore, or the weather will be atrocious. But remembering that deep motivation will push you out the door, even when all you want to do is sit on the couch.

I remember the first time I set a goal for myself. I was beginning my senior year of high school, and I wanted to win the state championship that year in cross country. I knew accomplishing that goal would take a lot of work and sacrifice, so I wrote the goal down and put it above my bed, in the gym, and any other place I could think of. That summer and fall, when I wanted to stay out late with friends, I remembered the goal. When I wanted to binge on chocolate sundaes, I remembered the goal. When the alarm went off at 5 a.m., I remembered the goal. And when October finally came around, I was in the best shape of my life. I accomplished the goal: I won that coveted state championship.

Looking back on it now, I'm still proud of that title. But what I'm prouder of (and what still impacts me to this day) is my dedication to the goal. Difficult goals require sacrifice, but the reward is always worth it.

Fun Runs

Although runners often talk about training for specific races and achieving certain times, it's important to remember that running should be fun. Sure, some days will be harder than others, but you should always feel satisfied when you finish a run—running should certainly never be anything you disdain. If you find yourself losing the joy of running, take a step back and focus on making running fun, again.

You can recapture the joy of running in a variety of ways. You can join a local running club or find a running partner, purchase a new running outfit, download a new podcast or playlist that keeps you excited, find a new trail or route to explore, or enter a "fun run" event: color runs, mud runs, inflatable runs, overnight relay races, murder mystery runs, midnight runs, costume runs. The list goes on and on, and new runs pop up all the time. To find one near you, check out the websites in the Resources section of this book.

Look to the Finish Line

As you think about and identify your goals, set realistic and achievable objectives.

Most new runners follow a similar trajectory. They start by trying to finish a few miles without feeling like they're going to pass out. Then they aim to finish their first 5k. Once they've had a taste of racing, they'll try a longer distance or see if they can run the next 5k a little faster. Eventually, most runners want to scale up in distance and try a half marathon (13.1 miles) and then a full marathon (26.2 miles).

This process—from beginner to first-time marathoner—should take about six months to a year. Avoid skipping too many steps in this trajectory. If you're just starting to run more seriously, it's going to be a monumental task to get ready for a marathon in a few months. The marathon can be your goal, but take smaller steps—such as racing a 5k first—to get to your ultimate destination.

Regardless of where you are in your journey, the plans in chapter 9 offer blueprints to help you achieve your goal. They will help you take the right steps, week by week, toward your ultimate objective.

Chart Your Progress

Whatever your goal, your focus should be on the process and the fundamentals. Focusing on the fundamentals means developing good habits, such as warming up before each run, getting in your technique and strength workouts each day, recovering properly, and executing your workouts. All these fundamentals will be covered in this book.

When I first started running, I read every magazine and book I could get my hands on. The next day, I'd try the "latest and greatest" workout I had just read about. After a few days, I'd feel like I wasn't getting any better,

so I'd search for the next magic formula. I toiled like this for months and actually started to race slower. Then my coach gave me a six-month fitness plan. I thought he was joking. The plan contained no fancy workouts, no jaw-dropping mileage—it was just consistent work, day after day. But I trusted him and followed the plan. Six months later, I was running better than I ever had. Since then, I've always trusted the process of long-term thinking. This consistent training won't impress people on social media, but it will ensure you make steady progress.

One strategy that helped me remain dedicated to the process was keeping a running log. I noted my workouts and how I felt after each one, which allowed me to look back over all my workouts at a glance. I looked at the log when my confidence in the plan wavered so I could see how far I'd come, even if I didn't feel like I had made any progress. This strategy helped me push past those bad workout days. I encourage you to start a running log as you use the workout plans in this book. You can keep a simple log in a notebook or you can use a tracking app on your phone, such as Strava or Runkeeper. Then, the next time you have doubts or you're enticed by a workout fad, you can see how far steady, consistent training has taken you.

How the Pros Stay Motivated

"Do elite runners ever lack motivation?"

I get asked this question a lot. The answer is a resounding "Yes!" Despite being incredibly good at what they do, elite runners suffer from the same doubts and struggles. Here are some inspirational quotes from pros on staying motivated:

"There are always going to be good and bad miles. If I'm in a bad one, I know there's a good one ahead."

—Amy Cragg, *champion marathon runner*

"You can still make something beautiful and something powerful out of a really bad situation."

—Gabe Grunewald, *national champion in the 3,000 meters*

"Only the disciplined ones are free in life. If you are undisciplined, you are a slave to your moods. You are a slave to your passions."

—Eliud Kipchoge, *Olympic marathon gold medalist*

"The battles that count aren't the ones for gold medals. The struggles within yourself—the invisible, inevitable battles inside all of us—that's where it's at."

—Jesse Owens, *four-time Olympic gold medalist*

"Some seek the comfort of their therapist's office, others head to the corner pub and dive into a pint, but I chose running as my therapy."

—Dean Karnazes, *world-renowned ultramarathon runner*

"You don't become a runner by winning a morning workout. The only true way is to marshal the ferocity of your ambition over the course of many days, weeks, months, and (if you could finally come to accept it) years. The Trial of Miles; Miles of Trials."

—John L. Parker Jr., *author of cult classic novel,* **Once a Runner**

"If you run, you are a runner. It doesn't matter how fast or how far. It doesn't matter if today is your first day or if you've been running for twenty years. There is no test to pass, no license to earn, no membership card to get. You just run."

—John Bingham, *marathon runner and author*

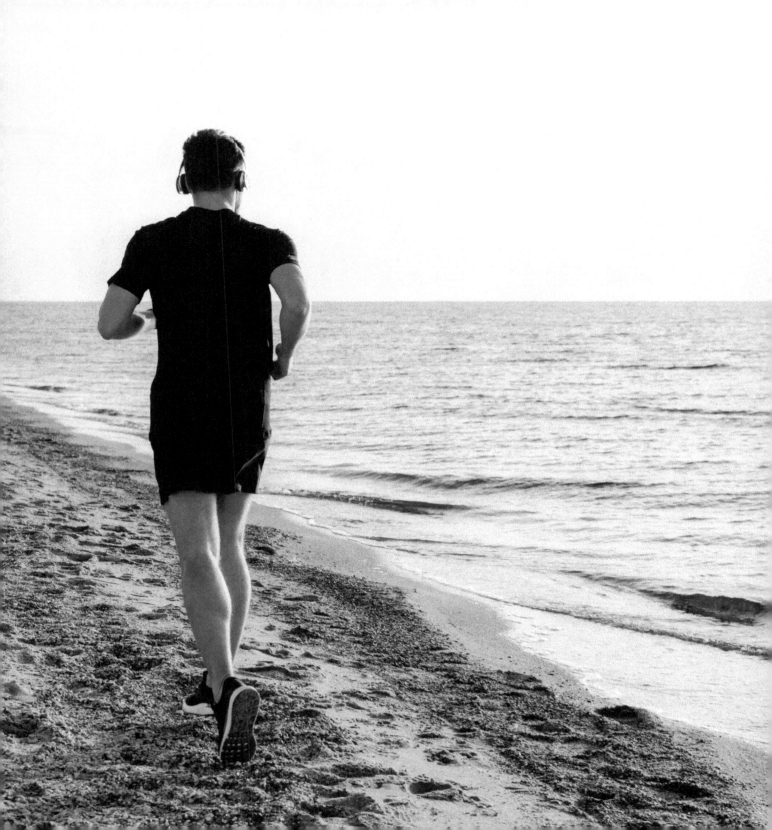

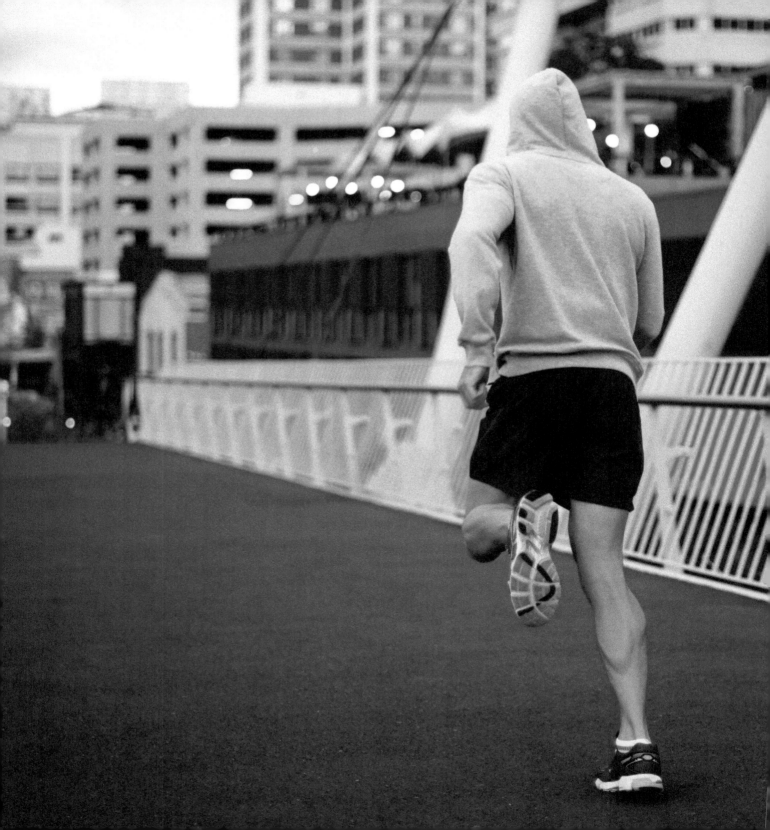

CHAPTER TWO

Dress Well, Run Well

One of the best ways to invest in your new running goals is to make sure you have the appropriate running gear—the correct shoes for your feet, appropriate clothing for the weather, and the right type of tracking devices to help you stay on target. These items may seem like an afterthought, but having great gear will help you stay injury-free and making consistent progress.

On Your Feet

Not surprisingly, the most important piece of running gear is your shoes. It's important you have a running shoe and not a shoe designed for cross-training or another sport. Running shoes are uniquely designed to provide the support and cushioning you need.

Everyone has a slightly different foot type and running motion. Running shoes are designed to help guide, correct, and support the way your foot naturally moves. It's important to select a shoe that supports the way your foot moves or you will only exacerbate any problems you have.

Your foot type is based on two factors. The first is *pronation*, a term used to describe how your foot moves when it first makes contact with the ground. A neutral pronation occurs when your foot lands just slightly on the outside and then rolls inward and pushes off the ground in a neutral position (or directly in the middle). *Overpronation* is when your foot rolls inward too much and your arch collapses, so that you take off from the inside of your foot, which leads to increased stress on your lower legs. *Underpronation*, also known as supination, is when the outside of your foot makes contact with the ground but your foot does not roll inward, which increases the amount of force that travels up your leg and can cause injuries, such as shin splints and stress fractures. Assessing pronation is difficult at home, but employees at your local running store should be able to determine your pronation by watching you walk or run.

The second factor for foot type is arch height. If, when standing barefoot, your arch collapses inward and there is no space between the floor and your foot, then you have a low or collapsing arch. If you have a significant amount of space between your arch and the floor, then you have a high arch.

To determine your arch type, you can do the "wet foot test." Simply wet the bottom of your foot and walk on a surface that will stay wet, such as a concrete floor or a piece of paper. You should see an imprint of your arch on the surface. If you barely see an imprint, then you have high arches. If the arch imprint is the same width as your foot, then you have low arches.

Another consideration for choosing running shoes is trail versus road. Trail and road shoes are the same in terms of pronation support and cushioning, but trail shoes are designed to be more water-resistant and have better traction. Unless you're doing a significant amount of running on technical trails with roots, climbs, and dirt, you should opt for a road shoe.

The Shoe Buyer's Checklist

Now that you understand why you need running shoes, it's time to head to the store. Here's a short checklist to help you choose the right shoe:

- [ ] Ask an employee to determine your arch type and pronation. These factors will narrow your selection to about a third of available shoes.

- [ ] Decide how much cushioning you want. There's no evidence that shoes with more cushioning prevent injuries better than ones with less cushioning. Choose what feels most comfortable for you.

- [ ] Double check your shoe size. Your running shoes will likely be a different size than your dress shoes. You should have a thumbnail-width space between the front of the shoe and your big toe.

- [ ] Try several brands to see which one fits your foot shape best. For the most part, all running shoe brands produce shoes of equal quality. The main difference is how the shoes fit. Some brands have wider toe boxes and are narrow in the heel, while others are made for runners with wide feet.

☐ Take your shoes for a test run around the store. Sometimes a shoe can feel slightly different when running instead of walking.

In Your Closet

Selecting the right clothes for your run is important. Choosing the right fabrics will prevent chafing and blisters, wick moisture, and keep you safe and comfortable in the elements. I highly recommend investing in your running wardrobe for long-term success. Few things demotivate a runner more than blisters or not having the right clothes for the weather.

Your Running Must-Haves

To help you get started, I've created some general guidelines for buying running attire.

I recommend that every article of clothing be made of moisture-wicking fabric. "Moisture-wicking" is a generic term for any fabric that self-dries and quickly moves (or wicks) sweat to the fabric's outer surface, so that your perspiration doesn't saturate the fabric. Cotton is not a moisture-wicking fabric and should be avoided for running attire, especially socks and underwear.

Every brand calls its moisture-wicking apparel by a different name but, generally speaking, the fabrics are made from the same synthetic materials. Every runner prefers one brand's apparel to another, so you may want to experiment with a few brands to find out which one you like best.

- Other than your shoes, socks are perhaps the most important purchase because they will help prevent blisters. When cotton socks get wet from perspiration, they rub against your skin, creating blisters. This is why you should opt for socks made from a moisture-wicking fabric.

- Pants or tights are important for cool mornings and for winter running. Loose pants or tights are a personal preference, but in either case, find a pair that fits well to reduce chafing.

- Shorts can be any length you feel comfortable in, but again, choose moisture-wicking fabrics that fit well to prevent chafing. You may have to experiment with a few brands to find the ones that fit you best.

- Underwear is often overlooked when runners select clothing. Most running shorts come with built-in support, so you may not always need underwear. However, most pants and tights do not, and you may find you prefer more support. Both men and women should look for moisture-wicking, breathable underwear.

- Avoid cotton shirts. When you sweat or when it rains, cotton will get heavy and uncomfortable. Cotton shirts will also keep you wet, which may make you cold during the second half of your run if it's raining or windy.

- The most important factor for a sports bra is fit. The band should be snug around your rib cage. You should be able to fit two fingers (but no more) between your body and the band. Wide bands tend to be more supportive than narrow bands.

- Jackets are important when it rains or if you run in cold environments. Running jackets are breathable and can repel some water. Depending on where you live, you may need one jacket for spring and fall and a different one for winter.

- Running hats and gloves or mittens are a must if you live in a cold climate. These items will wick your sweat away so you won't get too cold during the latter half of your runs.

Around Your Wrist

Today's high-tech running watches can perform many more tasks than the timepieces of yore—they really have much more in common with computers than watches. But with so many different kinds on the market, it can be overwhelming to choose.

Ultimately, it all comes down to how much data you want to track. My personal philosophy is only track data that you want to act on. Although it may be fun to collect 50 data points on each run, it might be difficult to glean the insights necessary to pinpoint what you need to work on.

Here's a quick cheat sheet to help you choose:

IF YOU WANT TO IMPROVE YOUR PACING . . .
. . . choose a watch with GPS to track your pace and distance.

IF YOU WANT TO BETTER JUDGE YOUR EFFORT . . .
. . . buy a heart-rate watch to keep track of your heart rate.

IF YOU WANT MORE FEEDBACK ON YOUR RUNNING MECHANICS . . .
. . . choose a stride-data watch, which collects data on elements such as cadence and stride length (see chapter 4 for more on these elements).

IF YOU JUST WANT TO GET OUT THERE AND RUN . . .
. . . go for the classic athletic wristwatch with a stopwatch.

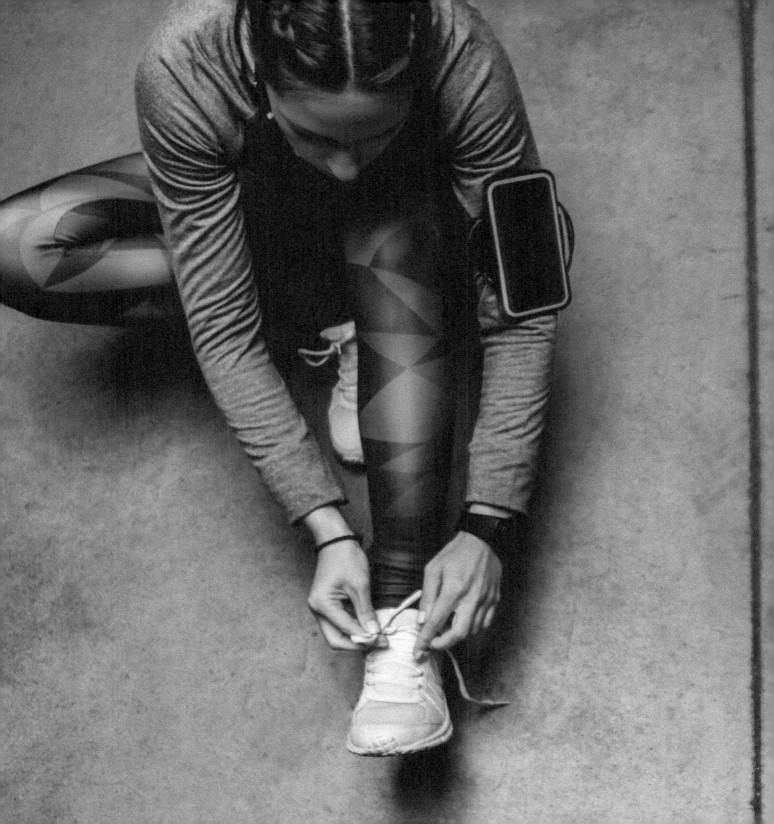

PART TWO

THE FUNDAMENTALS

Now that you have the mind-set and equipment you need to begin your running journey, it's time to discuss the fundamentals of running: proper running form and injury prevention. Understanding and establishing the fundamentals now will help you avoid injuries and make steady progress in the years to come.

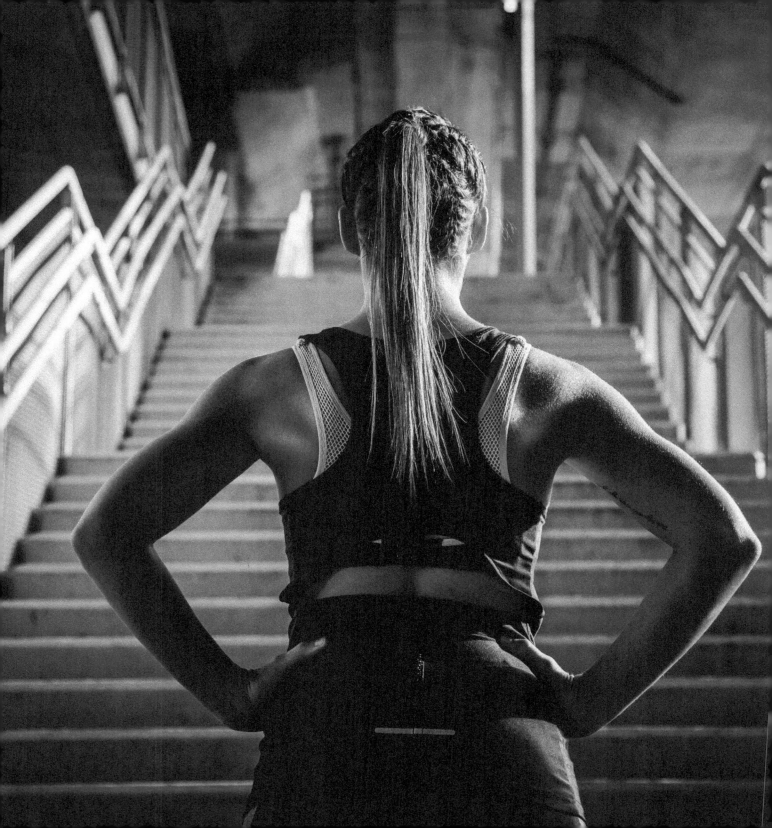

CHAPTER THREE

Posture and Alignment

Your running form is an interconnected chain of individual movements, much like cogs in a machine. The foundation of your form is your posture and alignment, so improving those components is the first step in developing a strong, efficient running stride.

In this chapter, you'll learn the basic elements of a strong running posture and alignment, why they're both critical to staying injury-free, and how to identify your own postural weaknesses through a series of simple tests you can perform at home.

Running Posture

Each element of your running form influences the other, but your posture holds it all together and affects every aspect.

Here's an example: If you are leaning backward when you run (as new runners commonly do), your glutes and hamstrings aren't in a strong enough position to properly fire. Since they can't generate enough force to power your stride, other muscles—such as your calves—need to take over and generate more force than they can handle. This poor running posture not only results in a less efficient stride, but can also cause calf strains and Achilles tendon injuries.

Proper running posture places your body in the most economical and powerful position for your unique stride, allowing all the elements of your running form to function efficiently.

The Basic Elements of Proper Running Posture

To help you better visualize your posture, it's helpful to break it down into the most important elements. The best way to analyze your posture is to have someone shoot a video of you running past the camera, and then coming straight toward it. You can take the video yourself by setting up a camera next to a treadmill. Once you have the video, take a closer look at the following:

Ankle Your ankle should be bent slightly forward as it travels underneath your body with each stride. This position will produce a slight forward lean.

Knee Your knee should track straight without collapsing inward when your foot is on the ground.

Pelvis Your pelvis should be in a neutral position, which means your two back hip points (the small bones you can feel to either side of your spine) should be on the same level as your pubic bones (the two bones you can feel in the front of your hip). If your back hip points are higher than your pelvis, you have an anterior pelvic tilt; if they are below your pelvis, you have a posterior pelvic tilt.

Shoulders Your shoulders should be held back. Your shoulder blades should be relaxed, if slightly contracted—not scrunched up toward your head. Think of running tall.

Head Your head position should be along the straight line that goes through your shoulder, hip, and the ball of your foot. You should not be craning your neck forward or back. Your eyes should be looking 30 to 40 feet in front of you.

How to Test Your Posture

These simple posture tests should be performed once a month to measure the progress of your exercises and training. If you fail any of the tests, do the Posture Routine (see page 21) in this chapter three to four times per week. If you pass these tests, do the routine two to three times per week.

The Knee Angle Test

Do three to five single-leg squats, keeping your torso upright and your knees about even with your toes. While you are doing these squats, glance down at your knee. Is it pointing straight ahead, or is it buckled or rotated inward? If your hip stabilizers are weak or if they aren't well coordinated, your knee will buckle inward.

The Pelvis Test

1. Lie on your back on the end of a table, so that you can hang off the edge without touching the ground. Your pelvis should be on the very edge of the table.

2. Pull one knee into your chest. Your other leg should be hanging freely in the air—not in contact with the ground.

3. Allow your down leg to relax and have a partner evaluate how far below the edge of the table your leg hangs. (If your leg is parallel, the thigh of your hanging leg is in a straight line with the table or your pelvis.)

4. If you don't have a partner, use your smartphone to take a 15- to 20-second delayed picture or video.

Determine your grade using the following criteria:

Poor: Your leg hangs above parallel with your body.

Average: Your leg hangs parallel with your body.

Good: Your leg hangs below parallel with your body.

The Vertical Compression Test

While you're in a standing position, have someone stand behind you and push straight down on your shoulders with moderate pressure. If your body buckles at the back and hips, your hips and balance may be off.

Running Alignment

In addition to posture, your rotational alignment is a critical piece of your running form. Rotational alignment refers to how your hips rotate with each stride. As your right leg moves forward, your hips will naturally rotate slightly to the right as your left arm comes forward to counterbalance. As you bring your right leg back and your left leg forward, your hips will rotate, again.

This slight rotation of the hips is natural, and it's a key element to staying healthy and driving your body forward. However, if you have excessive rotation at the hips, you can create increased tension within the pelvis, hips, and lower back. Conversely, if your hips do not rotate enough, you can't generate sufficient power from your stride, which often results in overstriding (see page 31).

The best way to "feel" your alignment is to imagine that your pelvis sits on a plane controlled by the two hip points in your back and the two points in the front of your pelvis. As you run, try not to allow your pelvis to tilt forward in either direction. Most runners find that they tilt their hips forward because they lack the strength and activation to fire their glutes properly. This tilting results in excessive hip rotation, as runners try to drive the leg backward.

Working Stiff

Most runners don't realize that everyday posture influences their stride. Unfortunately, many jobs require spending an inordinate amount of time sitting at a desk, in a car, or in front of a computer screen. The result: Our hip flexors and hamstrings are constantly placed in a shortened position, which inevitably tightens them up and makes it harder for them to move through the range of motion necessary to run properly.

Many people slouch when sitting in front of a computer—it's practically human nature. With our shoulders rounded so often, the spine's ability to rotate and extend fully becomes limited. Without that full range of motion in our midsection, we can't properly rotate our hips.

Here are a few strategies you can use at work to combat the negative effects of sitting too much, and keep your posture in check.

Use a standing desk. Switch to a standing desk, if you can. Even 15 or 30 minutes a day can begin to improve your posture and overall health.

Sit on a stability ball. Switch out your regular office chair for a stability ball to activate your core. Start by using it 5 to 10 minutes every hour and slowly build up your tolerance.

Go for a walk. Set an alarm as a reminder to get up and move every hour. Walk for three minutes, stretch a little, or do a few lunges. It might look funny to bystanders, but trust me, the benefit is worth it.

Perform dynamic stretches. Use the second half of your lunch break or any other 10- or 15-minute period to perform the dynamic stretches from the next section of this chapter. You don't have to complete an entire routine—just focus on the areas that are the tightest. Not only will these routines improve your runs, but they'll increase your blood flow, making you more productive at work.

Posture Routine (PR)

The following routine is a simple yet effective technique for improving your running posture. The routine only takes a few minutes to complete, so it's easy to add to your training schedule either before or after your run. I've added this routine to the training plans in chapter 9. If you're creating your own plan, implement the posture routine two or three days per week, ideally after an easy run.

STRETCH NAME	INSTRUCTIONS
Standing Crescent Moon	Hold 15 seconds, each side
Wide-Legged Forward Fold with Chest Expansion	Hold 10 seconds
Kneeling Lat	Hold 15 seconds
Supine Spinal Twist	Hold 3 seconds each side, 10 each side
Open-Heart Stretch	Hold 3 seconds, 10 repetitions

STANDING CRESCENT MOON

Area worked: Obliques

1. Stand tall with your feet shoulder-width apart. Hold your right hand high above your head and keep your left hand relaxed by your side.

2. Exhale. Press your right hip out to the right side, arching your upper torso to the left. Keep your feet grounded and continue to reach up with your right hand.

3. Hold for 15 seconds. Return to the starting position and repeat with the opposite side.

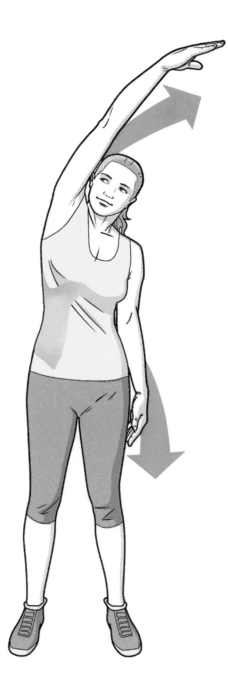

WIDE-LEGGED FORWARD FOLD WITH CHEST EXPANSION

Areas worked: Inner thighs, chest, and back

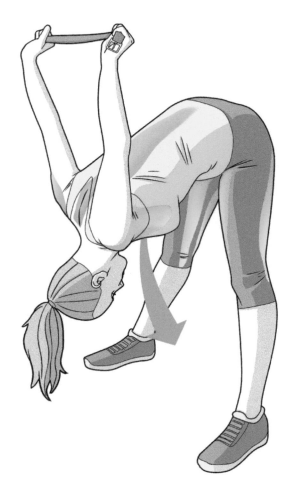

1. Start in a standing position with your legs two or three feet wider than shoulder-width. Your arms should be behind you, and you should be holding a small towel or washcloth.

2. Bend down at the waist while bringing your arms up behind you. Stop when your upper body is just below your waist. Your arms should be straight out behind you, as parallel with the ground as possible.

3. Hold this position for 10 seconds.

KNEELING LAT

Area worked: Lats

1. Kneel in front of a chair with the seat facing you.

2. Bend over and extend your arms so that your forearms rest comfortably on the chair when your arms are fully extended. Adjust your body's distance from the chair as needed.

3. Keeping your shoulders and arms straight, supported by the seat of the chair, inhale and press your chest toward the ground. You should feel the stretch on your sides.

4. Hold this position for 15 seconds.

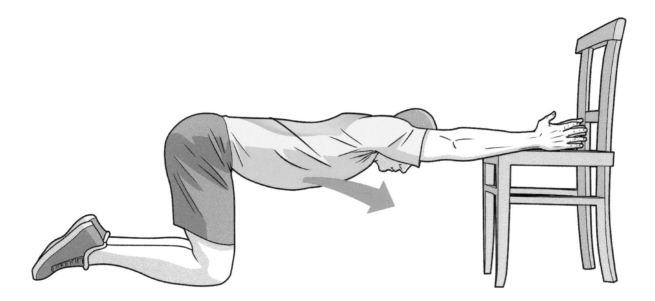

SUPINE SPINAL TWIST

Areas worked: Lower back, hips, and glutes

1. Lying on your back, bring your arms out to the sides with the palms facing down in a T position. Bend your right knee and place your right foot on your left knee.

2. Exhale and move your right knee over to the left side of your body, twisting your spine and lower back. Turn your head and look toward your right fingertips.

3. Keep your shoulders flat to the floor, close your eyes, and soften into the posture. Let gravity pull your knee down. You should not have to use any effort in this posture.

4. Breathe in and out. Hold the position for 3 seconds.

5. Inhale as you begin to release the position and roll your hips back to the floor. Exhale while you move your leg back down to the floor.

6. Repeat on the other side.

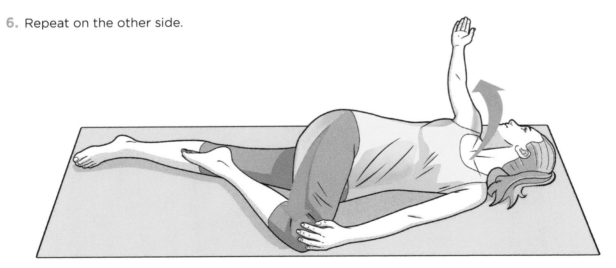

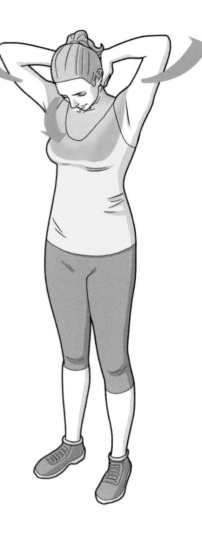

OPEN-HEART STRETCH

Areas worked: Chest and upper back

1. Stand tall with your hands interlaced behind the back of your head.

2. Lean your neck and elbows forward, almost so you're slouching, bringing your chin to your chest.

3. Flex your elbows, neck, and chest backward. Concentrate on getting as much of a stretch as you can from your chest. It should feel like you're reaching back with your elbows.

4. Hold for 3 to 5 seconds. This is one repetition.

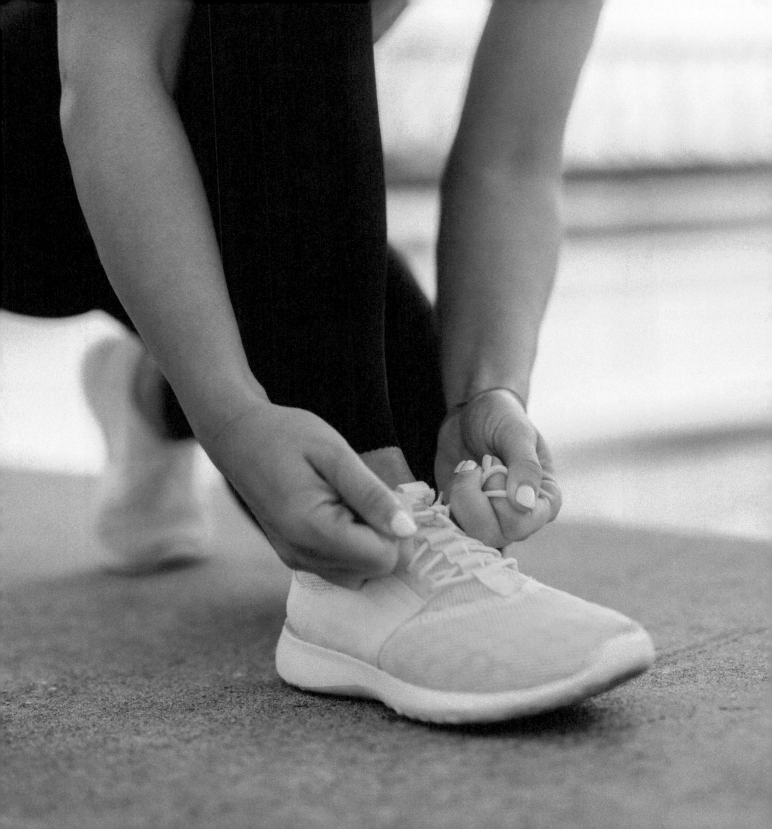

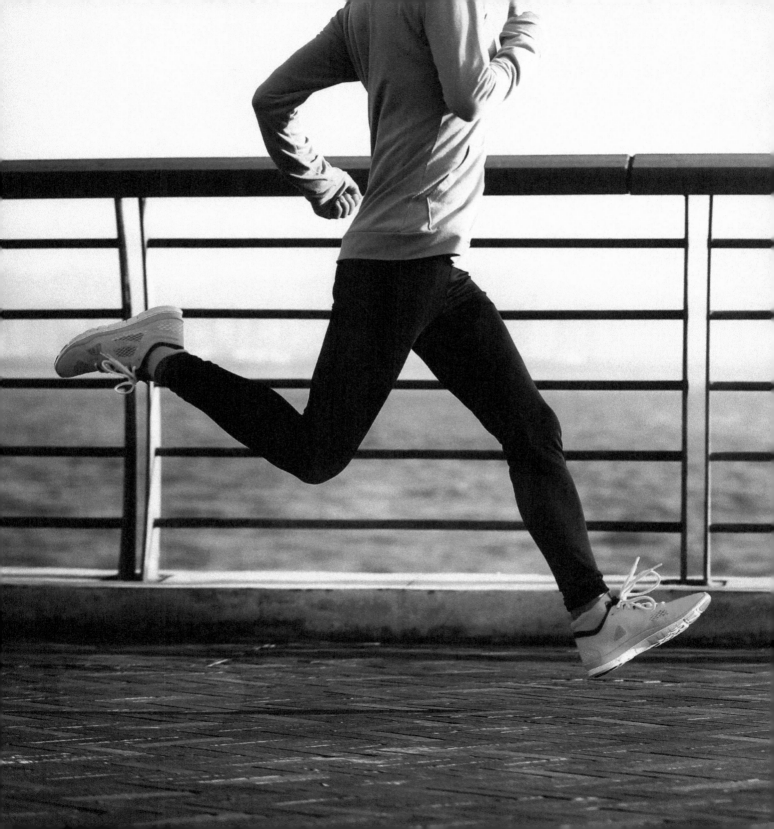

CHAPTER FOUR

Mastering Your Stride

Runners and coaches use the term "stride" to define the movements your legs make when you're running. As you'll learn in this chapter, your stride is composed of many different moving parts. The goal of this chapter is to help you understand the elements of your stride so you can make safe, effective improvements.

Running Stride

There is no optimal stride that works for every runner. Your optimal stride is going to be one-of-a-kind because your body is unique. Maybe you have wide hips and short legs; maybe you have a short Achilles tendon or inflexibility in your back that prevents a full range of motion. Either way, your stride is never going to look the same as that of your running partner or any of the elites you see on TV. That's perfectly fine—embrace it!

Part of learning to love your stride is finding your optimal stride based on your body type and areas of strength and weakness. Often, this stride is called *self-selected stride*. To achieve it, you have to fix the things that impede your body from moving the way it was meant to—such as tight or weak muscles. Improving your stride doesn't mean trying to emulate another runner or consciously trying to change it as you run. Improving your stride means strengthening personal areas of weakness so that those parts will perform their roles when you run.

Here are some relevant terms to help you better understand your stride. Later in this chapter, I'll introduce some simple stretches to help you make improvements.

Stride length This is the distance covered between each step you take. If you take off or push forward with your right leg, stride length is the distance you travel before your left leg touches the ground. Your stride length will naturally get longer as you run faster and shorter when you run slower. Some wearable devices will measure your stride length, but this element is not something you should actively try to change.

Cadence This is how fast you move your legs. Cadence is usually measured in steps per minute. To determine your cadence, count the number of times your left foot hits the ground for 30 seconds. Double that to get the total for 60 seconds, then double it again to get the total for both feet.

Stance phase The stance phase is composed of the moments during your stride when your foot is on the ground. The phase starts when your foot initially touches the ground (initial contact), goes through when your foot is directly under you and supporting all your weight (midstance), and ends when your leg starts to propel you forward (propulsion).

Swing phase The swing phase describes the motion of your leg when it is off the ground. This phase starts when your heel begins to lift toward your buttocks, moves forward as your leg swings under your hips, and ends as your leg unfolds before your foot touches the ground.

The Tendency to Overstride

Overstriding is the most common and critical mistake runners make. Overstriding is when your foot lands out in front of your body, typically with a straight or only slightly bent leg. When your foot lands this way, your leg can't properly absorb the shock of hitting the ground, and the impact travels up and into your knees and hips—a common cause of injury.

Overstriding can be caused by a variety of factors. Here are a few of the primary culprits:

1. If your hip flexors are tight, you don't generate enough hip extension to swing your leg forward fast enough to get under your body.

2. If you lean back, your body shifts back as well, making it nearly impossible to get your leg directly under you.

3. When newer runners attempt to run faster, they reach out with their legs to try and increase their stride length.

These examples all illustrate one principle: It's unwise—and unsafe—to consciously try to change your stride. The causes of overstriding likely stem from a lack of mobility or strength somewhere in your body. Trying to change the way you run will only lead to another problem as your body attempts to compensate. The best way to improve your stride is to eliminate areas of inflexibility and weakness with stretching and strength training.

Stride On

Although each runner's self-selected stride differs, there are some guiding principles for a strong running stride. You may notice these principles are similar to the elements of proper running posture, but I think they're worth reinforcing in this context.

1. Your head should be in a relaxed, neutral position, meaning it's not tilted left or right and you're not leaning forward or backward. You should be looking about 30 to 40 feet in front of you.

2. Your shoulders should be as relaxed as possible, not hunched up toward your neck or ears.

3. Your upper body should lean slightly forward, from the ankles, to help generate proper extension at the hip.

4. Your arms should be relaxed and swinging to facilitate forward motion. Don't swing them side to side. Your elbows should be bent and only move slightly with each stride. Your thumbs should graze your hips.

5. Your hips should be in a neutral position (not tilted forward or backward). With each stride, your leg should extend backward to capitalize on the elastic energy contained in the hip flexors.

6. Your leg should land directly or almost directly under your body (your center of mass) with a slight bend at the knee.

The Foot Strike Conundrum

The term "foot strike" refers to your foot's position as it first touches the ground with each stride. There are three ways your foot can hit the ground:

Heel strike (rearfoot) This refers to when your heel contacts the ground first, followed by the rest of your foot. This type of foot strike is the most common type.

Midfoot strike This is when you first contact the ground with the entire center of your foot. Usually, you strike slightly on the outside first and roll inward.

Forefoot strike This occurs when you land on the ball of your foot. Often, with this kind of strike, the heel never touches the ground.

A wealth of recent research has indicated that there is no ideal foot strike. Scientists and coaches used to believe that landing with a heel strike led to most running injuries. However, studies have since proven that it's not the heel strike that leads to the injuries, but rather the fact that all runners who overstride *also* heel strike—it's the overstriding that leads to the injuries. Ultimately, if you heel strike but don't overstride—meaning your foot lands under your body—then you still have a safe and efficient foot strike.

Stride Routine (SR)

This simple routine will help you develop the flexibility and strength to eliminate your inhibitions and achieve your self-selected stride. Each exercise was chosen to alleviate the most common problems runners have with their strength and mobility. The routine only takes a few minutes to complete, so it's easy to add to your training schedule either before or after you run. I've added this routine to the sample training plans in chapter 9. If you're creating your own plan, implement the Stride Routine two or three days per week, preferably after a hard workout or a long run.

STRETCH NAME	INSTRUCTIONS
Supported Low Lunge	Hold 15 seconds, each side
Downward-Facing Dog	Hold 10 seconds
Ankle Circles	10 each direction, each leg
Reverse Tabletop	Hold 10 seconds
Glutes Stretch	Hold 10 seconds, each leg

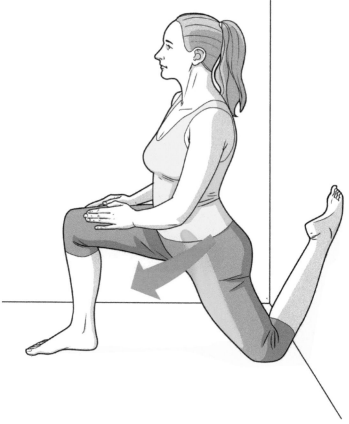

SUPPORTED LOW LUNGE

Area worked: Hip flexors

1. Kneel on your left knee with your left foot braced against a wall and your right foot directly in front of you.

2. Slowly lean forward, stretching your left hip toward the floor.

3. Hold for 15 seconds.

4. Switch sides and repeat.

BEGINNER TIP: Remember to squeeze your glutes, which will allow you to stretch your hip flexor even more.

DOWNWARD-FACING DOG

Areas worked: Calves and hamstrings

1. Start on your hands and feet with your buttocks in the air. Keep your arms and legs straight with your wrists in line with your shoulders and your toes tucked.

2. Keeping your arms and legs straight, slowly walk your legs forward until you feel a good stretch. Don't overdo it.

3. Take a deep breath and press your heels and arms into the ground. This movement should increase the stretch in your calves and upper back.

4. Hold for 10 seconds and release.

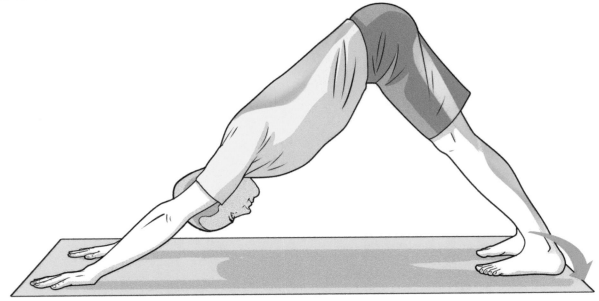

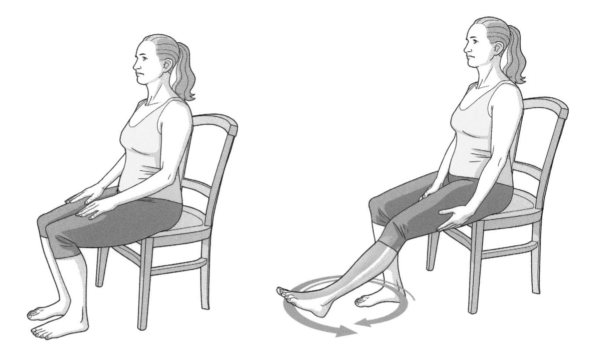

ANKLE CIRCLES

Areas worked: Ankles, calves, and feet

1. Start by sitting in a chair and lifting one foot slightly off the ground.

2. Slowly move your foot in a circular motion. Try to extend your foot and ankle as far in each direction as you can.

3. Perform 10 circles in one direction, then reverse direction and perform 10 more.

REVERSE TABLETOP

Areas worked: Chest, glutes, lower back, and quads

1. Start by sitting on your buttocks, knees bent, with your arms on the floor behind you and your palms facing forward.

2. Inhale, lifting your hips while pressing firmly onto your hands and feet. Straighten your arms. Make sure your knees are at a 90-degree angle and your thighs and torso are parallel to the floor. Your wrists should be directly underneath your shoulders.

3. Move your shoulder blades close to each other and open your chest. Hold for 10 seconds. You can keep your neck neutral, or you can gently begin to drop your head if that feels comfortable for your neck.

BEGINNER TIP: Relax the glutes and keep the pose using only the strength of your legs.

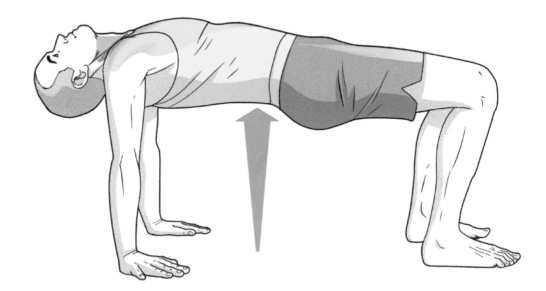

GLUTES STRETCH

Areas worked: Glutes, hips, and piriformis

1. Start by lying flat on your back with both knees bent.

2. Put your left leg on top of the other knee. Your left leg should now be perpendicular to your right. Your left knee and right knee should be on the same plane, with your shinbone connecting them.

3. Slowly begin to lift your right leg toward your chest. Make sure your left knee stays in-line with your left knee. Don't let your knee drop.

4. Stop when you feel the stretch in your hips and glutes.

5. Hold for 10 seconds and then switch legs.

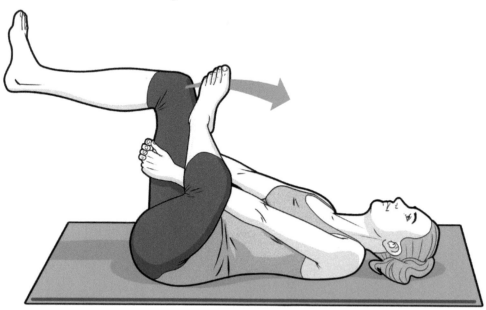

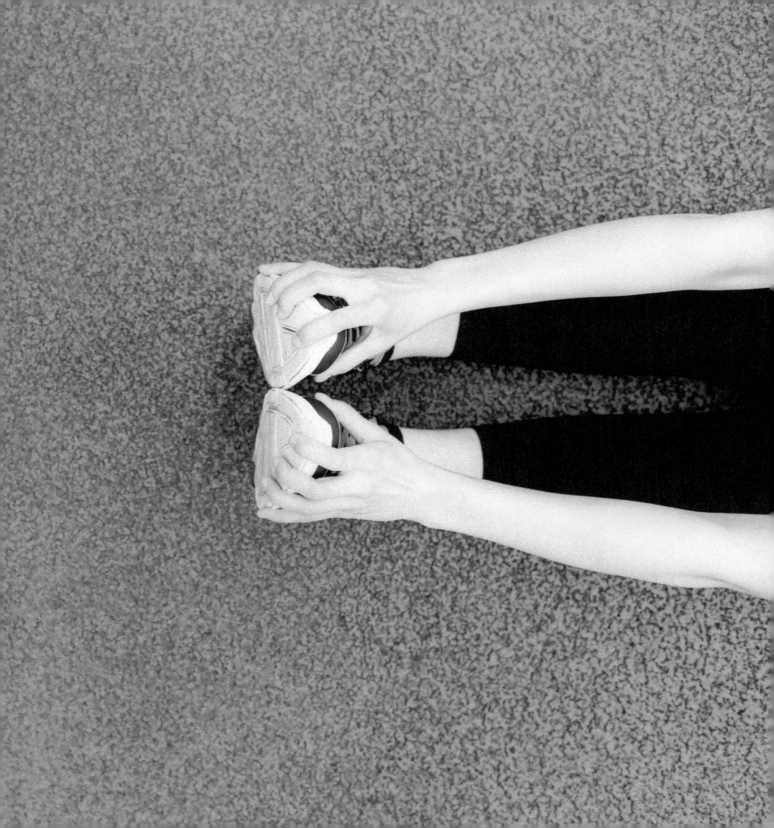

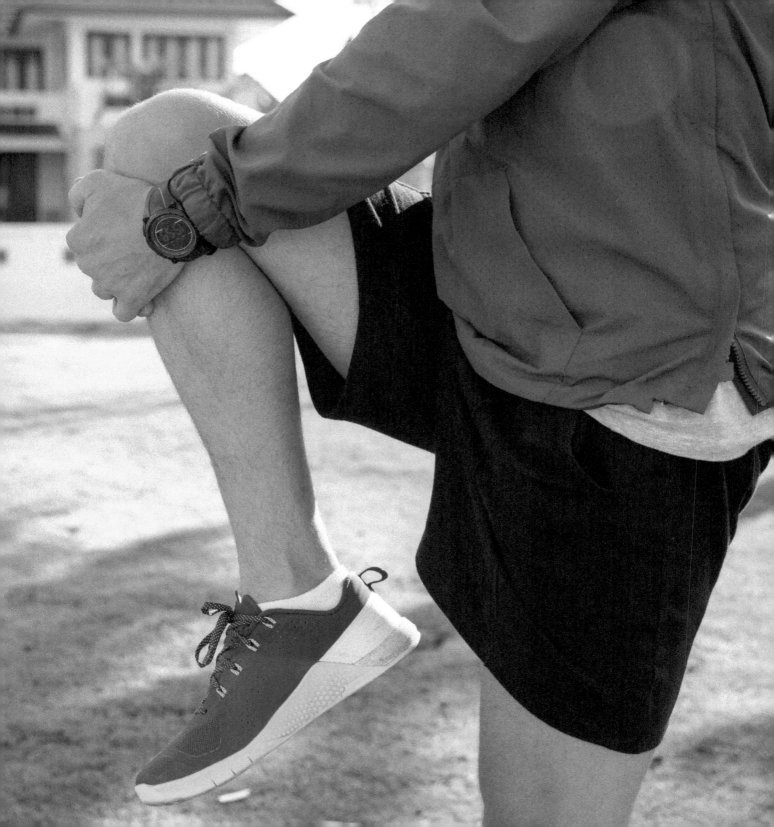

CHAPTER FIVE

Warm-Up, Recovery, and Injury Prevention

Any serious runner risks getting injured. In fact, recent research has shown that as many as 79 percent of runners are injured at least once a year (van Gent et al. 2007). You can greatly reduce your chances of contributing to that statistic by creating a total-body running plan. Research has shown that a running plan that includes proper strength work, stretching, and form drills can help keep you injury-free. In this chapter, I'll outline some of that research and give you routines to properly warm up, cool down, recover, and prevent injuries.

Why We Stretch

As you learned in chapters 3 and 4, stretching can help correct your posture and improve your form. Stretching after a run also helps avoid injuries. A 2005 study of athletes with hamstring injuries showed that implementing a post-run stretching routine reduced the instance of injuries by nearly 70 percent (Verrall et al. 2005).

Stretching before your workout is critical to warming up because it increases blood flow to your muscles and activates them in preparation for a run. The type of stretching you want to do before a run is called *Active Isolated Stretching* (AIS).

AIS involves stretching the targeted area for two to three seconds, releasing the stretch, relaxing, and then returning to stretching. AIS typically involves some assistance with a rope or your hands. The theory behind AIS is that, after two or three seconds, a muscle will begin to contract, which negates the benefits of the stretch. By releasing every two or three seconds, you avoid this contraction phase. This movement pattern is also why AIS is perfect for pre-run stretching: It helps increase blood flow before your run.

Of course, stretching after your run is important as well. When you run, your muscles get stiff and shorten to protect themselves from injury. When you don't properly stretch after your run, the muscles remain in this shortened state. Soon, they'll lack the mobility to maintain proper running form. After your run, you can employ AIS or *static stretching*, the type of stretching in which you hold a stretch for 5 to 15 seconds.

In this chapter, I provide two stretching routines. Try to complete the AIS routine before every run. It is especially crucial to perform this type of stretching before harder or faster running days. If you don't properly warm up and stretch before faster workout days, you're significantly more vulnerable to injury. As for after your run, research suggests that AIS is superior; however, depending on your preference, you can choose the static or AIS.

Flexibility vs. Mobility

You may hear people use "mobility" and "flexibility" interchangeably, but it's important to understand the difference between the two. Flexibility refers to the ability of your muscles to stretch. Mobility, on the other hand, is how easily an area of your body can move through its entire range of motion.

Although flexibility is beneficial, mobility is more important for runners: If your muscles can't move through their entire range of motion, it doesn't matter how flexible they are—your stride is going to be inhibited. Flexibility is best targeted with static stretching, whereas mobility is best targeted with AIS.

Static Stretching Routine (SS)

This routine includes five essential static stretches for runners. Depending on your preference, you can perform either this routine or the AIS routine (see page 49) after your run.

STRETCH NAME	INSTRUCTIONS
Bound Angle	Hold 15 seconds
Thread the Needle	Hold 3 seconds each side, 10 each side
Quad Stretch	Hold 15 seconds, each leg
Standing Calf Stretch	Hold 15 seconds, each leg
Glutes Stretch	Hold 10 seconds, each leg

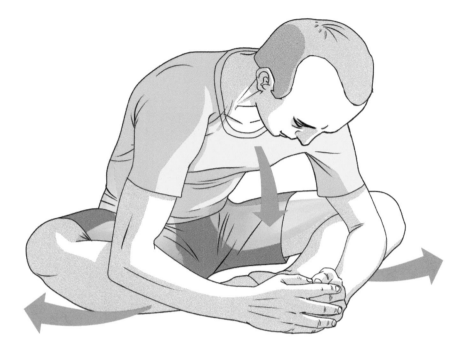

BOUND ANGLE

Areas worked: Groin, hips, inner thighs, and lower back

1. Sit up tall with the soles of your feet pressed together and your knees dropped to the sides as far as they will comfortably go.

2. Pull your abdominals gently inward and lean forward from your hips.

3. Grasp your feet with your hands and carefully pull yourself a little farther forward.

4. Hold for 15 seconds. Increase the stretch by carefully pressing your thighs toward the floor.

THREAD THE NEEDLE

Areas worked: Lower back, shoulders, and upper back

1. Begin on your hands and knees. Your wrists should be directly under your shoulders and your knees directly under your hips with your fingertips pointed toward the top of your mat. Center your head in a neutral position and soften your gaze downward.

2. On an exhalation, slide your right arm underneath your left arm with your palm facing up. Let your right shoulder come all the way down to the mat. Rest your right ear and cheek on the mat, then gaze toward your left.

3. Keep your left elbow lifted and your hips raised. Do not press your weight onto your head. Adjust your position so you do not strain your neck or shoulder.

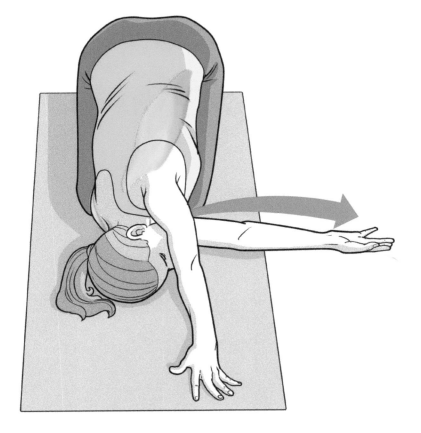

4. Let your upper back broaden. Soften and relax your lower back. Allow all the tension in your shoulders, arms, and neck to drain away.

5. Hold for 3 seconds. To release, press through your left hand and gently slide your right hand out. Return to the start and prepare to repeat on the other side.

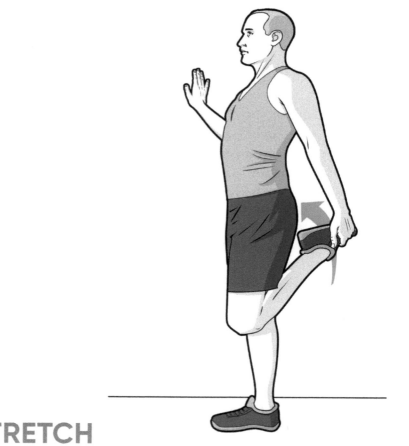

QUAD STRETCH

Area worked: Quads

1. Stand tall with your feet hip-width apart, pull your abdominals in, and relax your shoulders.

2. Bend your left leg, bringing your heel toward your buttocks, and grasp your left foot with your hand.

3. Hold for 15 seconds and then repeat with the other leg.

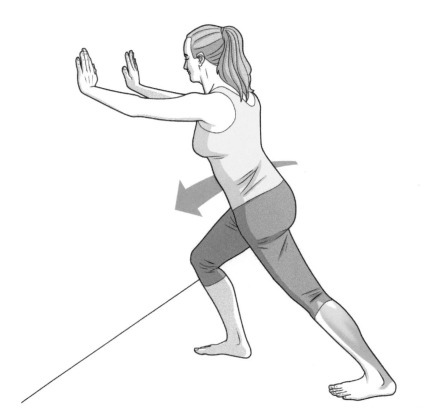

STANDING CALF STRETCH

Area worked: Calves

1. Stand facing the wall with your arms straight out in front of you.

2. Step your right leg forward and lean so that your hands are braced against the wall. Keep your left leg semi-straight.

3. Hold for 15 seconds. You should feel the stretch in your left calf. Lean forward a bit more to increase the stretch. Then switch sides.

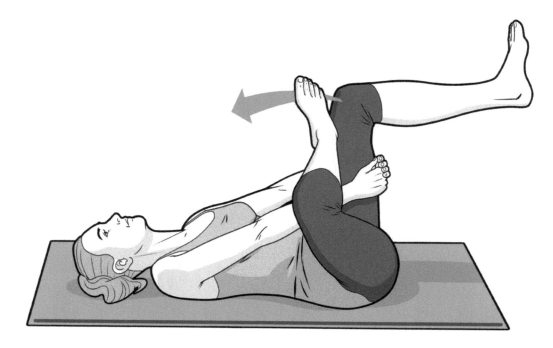

GLUTES STRETCH

Areas worked: Glutes, hips, and piriformis

1. Start by lying flat on your back with both knees bent.

2. Put your right leg on top of the other knee. Your right leg should now be perpendicular to your left. Your right knee and left knee should be in the same plane, with your shinbone connecting them.

3. Slowly begin to lift your left leg toward your chest. Make sure your right knee stays in line with your left knee. Don't let your knee drop.

4. Stop when you feel the stretch in your hips and glutes.

5. Hold for 10 seconds and then switch legs.

AIS Routine (AS)

These five essential AIS stretches for runners make a suitable pre-run stretching routine. You can perform this routine after your run as well.

STRETCH NAME	INSTRUCTIONS
Assisted Supine Hamstring Stretch	10 repetitions, each leg
Piriformis Stretch	10 repetitions, each leg
AIS Calf Stretch	10 repetitions, each leg
Supine Spinal Twist	Hold 3 seconds, 10 each side
Ankle Circles	10 each direction, each leg

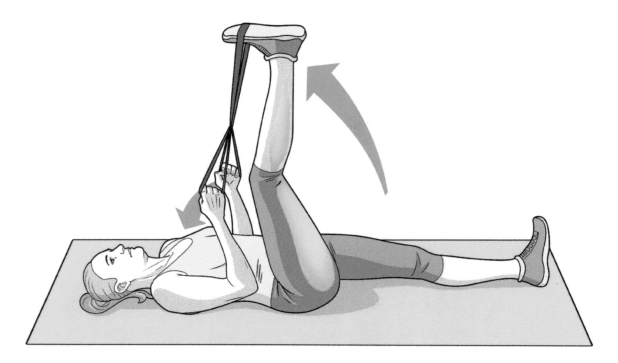

ASSISTED SUPINE HAMSTRING STRETCH

Area worked: Hamstrings

1. Lie on the floor with your legs extended in front of you. Loop an elastic band or towel around the ball of one foot.

2. Raise your leg by pulling the band toward you while keeping your knee straight.

3. Pull the band until you feel a stretch in your hamstring.

4. Hold for 3 seconds, then release and relax your hamstring. This is one repetition.

5. Repeat step 3. Try to take your leg back a little farther with each repetition.

PIRIFORMIS STRETCH

Areas worked: Hips, piriformis, and glutes

1. Start by lying flat on your back with both knees bent.

2. Put your right leg on top of the other knee. Your right leg should now be perpendicular to your left. Your right knee and left knee should be on the same plane, with your shinbone connecting them.

3. Slowly begin to lift your left leg toward your chest. Make sure your right knee stays in line with your left knee. Don't let your knee drop.

4. Stop and hold for 3 seconds when you feel the stretch in your hips and glutes. This is one repetition.

5. Relax the leg and then repeat step 3. Try to take your leg back slightly farther with each repetition.

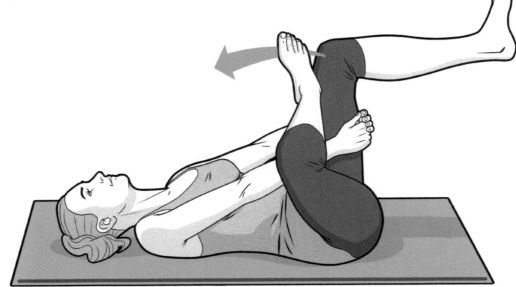

AIS CALF STRETCH

Area worked: Calves

1. Sit with both legs straight out in front of you.

2. Loop an elastic band or a towel around the ball of your left foot.

3. From your heel, flex your foot back toward your ankle, using the rope for a gentle assist at the end of the movement.

4. Stop and hold for 3 seconds when you feel the stretch in your calf. This is one repetition.

5. Relax the leg and then repeat step 3. Try to take your foot back a little farther with each repetition.

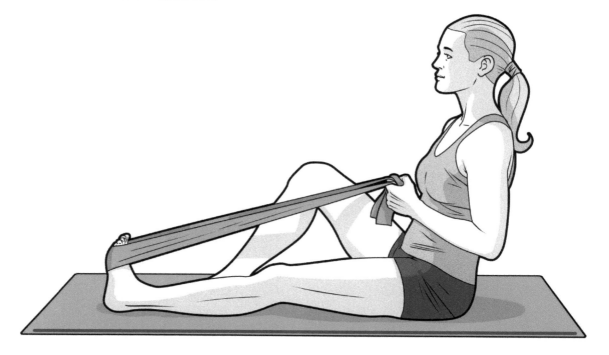

SUPINE SPINAL TWIST

Areas worked: Lower back, hips, and glutes

1. Lying on your back, bring your arms out to your sides with the palms facing down in a T position. Bend your right knee and place your right foot on your left knee.

2. Exhale and move your right knee over to the left side of your body, twisting your spine and lower back. Turn your head and look toward your right fingertips.

3. Keep your shoulders flat to the floor, close your eyes, and soften into the posture. Let gravity pull your knee down. You should not have to use any effort in this posture.

4. Breathe in and out. Hold the position for 3 seconds. This is one repetition.

5. Inhale as you begin to release the position and roll your hips back to the floor. Exhale while you move your leg back down to the floor.

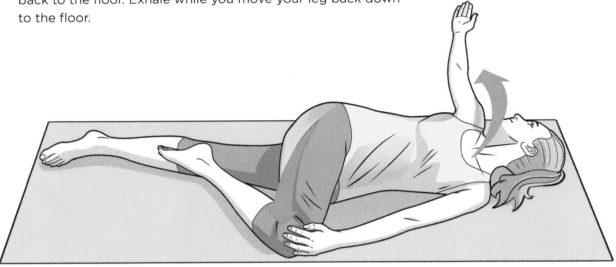

ANKLE CIRCLES

Areas worked: Ankles, calves, and feet

1. Start by sitting in a chair and lifting one foot slightly off the ground.

2. Slowly move your foot in a circular motion. Try to extend your foot and ankle as far in each direction as you can.

3. Perform 10 circles in one direction, then reverse direction and perform 10 more.

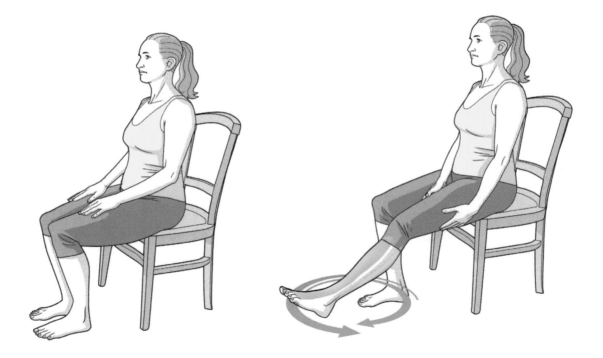

How Running Injuries Happen

Running injuries primarily occur for two reasons: structural issues, such as having a weakness in a certain area or not having the mobility to run with proper form, and improper training, such as running hard every day or increasing your weekly mileage too quickly. In chapters 6 and 7, I offer ways to fix structural problems. In chapters 8 and 9, I concentrate on giving you the right guidance to train injury-free.

Running injuries may be classified in a few different ways. Understanding the root of the injury will help you address the cause.

Overload injuries These injuries happen when a specific muscle or area of the body tries to do more work than it's capable of. An example of this is a calf strain. The problem stems from the fact that your calf is being required to produce more force (or contract more forcefully) than it's ready to. Although the pain might be in your calf, the problem may originate in your hips and glutes. Due to poor posture, your hips and glutes may not be generating enough power, leaving your calf to pick up the slack.

Overuse injuries Overuse injuries generally occur when you don't give your body enough time to recover or when you progress your training too quickly. Running is a sport that requires performing the exact same movements hundreds, even thousands, of times each day. It's not surprising that some injuries are the result of this repetition.

Chronic injuries Usually, these injuries slowly get worse over time. The pain may start out as a dull annoyance, but as you continue to train, the pain can become almost debilitating. A good example of this type of injury is plantar fasciitis, where the tendon that connects your toes to your heel slowly detaches itself from the heel. Initially, the pain is only slight, but the more you aggravate the injury, the worse it becomes. The key to preventing chronic injuries is to treat them as soon as you start to feel any pain. If you catch the injury in its early stages, it can be an easy fix. If you wait until the injury is full-blown, you may not be able to run for months.

Compensation injuries These injuries are very common for runners who try to return to running too soon after an injury. They typically progress like this: One area of your body is still sore from a previous injury, resulting in a slight limp. Consequently, another part of your body must compensate for the still-injured area, leading to yet another injury in the part of the body doing the compensating. It's a vicious cycle. Always be cautious when returning from injuries!

What to Do If You Get Injured

At some point, no matter what you do, its likely an injury will occur. Even elite runners with teams of physicians and trainers at their disposal aren't spared. If you are injured, here are a few steps to help you get back on the road as quickly as possible.

1. Stop running! It probably sounds obvious, but this is the most crucial piece of advice any coach could give you. Trying to run through an injury will only make it worse.

2. Start a treatment plan as soon as possible. A treatment plan involves stretching, massaging, and strength work. It may also include physical therapy, depending on the severity of the injury.

3. If the injury is serious and requires the assistance of a medical professional, find a good physical therapist or sports doctor in your area. If you're not sure who to see, try visiting the local running shop or asking your experienced running friends for a recommendation. A physical therapist will help you develop a recovery plan. And remember: use icing and anti-inflammatories sparingly. These old-school treatments can actually delay healing, because inflammation is the body's natural way to treat injuries.

4. Don't slack on the injury-prevention work and cross-training (see page 78). A lot of runners get down when they can't run and stop doing anything active. You can still make progress while cross-training, and injury-prevention work will help you get back on the road faster.

5. When getting back out there, follow these two simple rules:

   A. You shouldn't have pain when walking or cross-training. If you have pain, your injury isn't healed.
   B. It's okay if there is a little soreness after you run, but the soreness should not worsen each day.

A Post-Run Injury-Prevention Routine

As with your overall health, prevention is the best medicine for running injuries, because most running injuries are caused by a lack of strength or mobility. If you can improve your strength and mobility before injuries happen, you can avoid injuries altogether. For example, a study conducted at Stanford University in 2000 showed that implementing a hip injury-prevention routine reduced the chances of contracting IT band syndrome (one of the most common running injuries) by 91 percent (Fredericson 2000).

To help you stay injury-free, I've put together this simple post-run injury-prevention routine. You should implement this routine after every run. In total, it will take 15 to 20 minutes, but the long-term benefits will help you stay injury-free and become a more well-rounded runner. Here's how it works:

1. Finish your run and get hydrated. You can have water or a sports beverage, but aim to drink six to eight ounces of fluid to replenish what you lost during the run.

2. Perform a post-run stretching routine. This cool-down activity could be the AIS Routine (see page 49) or the Static Stretching Routine (see page 43) mentioned earlier in this chapter, or the Posture Routine (see page 21) or Stride Routine (see page 33) mentioned in chapters three and four.

3. Start your strength training or drill work. Follow one of the sample training plans in chapter 9 or consult chapters 6 and 7 to learn how to implement these exercises on your own.

4. Refuel with carbohydrates and protein. Chocolate milk, yogurt and granola, or a banana and peanut butter on a bagel are excellent choices. Aim for a four-to-one ratio of carbohydrates to protein.

Remember to Recover

As a competitive runner, I know it's tempting to train harder, run farther, and keep pushing your limits. But in order to improve as a runner, building recovery in to your training is essential. In fact, I'd argue that recovery is actually more important than the hard work you put into improving as a runner.

Getting fitter and stronger happens because when you run or do strength work, you break down and slightly tear your muscle fibers, which is why you get sore and tired after a hard workout. When you rest, your body starts to repair these damaged muscles. Your body even tries to build the muscles back stronger, because it wants to be better prepared next time you go for a run. This process is how and why you're able to gain strength and get faster, week after week, month after month.

Unfortunately, if you don't give your body enough time to rest and recover between hard workouts, your body can't repair your damaged muscles. You simply continue to accumulate damage. You may be able to stand to push through for a few days or a week, but eventually your body is going to break down and you're going to overtrain—or, worse, suffer an injury.

How to Recover

Every running plan should include ample recovery and rest. This recovery can come in multiple forms.

Between runs All the training plans in chapter 9 include rest days and cross-training to give your legs a break from pounding the pavement. Your strength training and drill days are also spaced out so that you're not working the same areas two or three days in a row.

Sleeping It's critical that as you increase your training, you get adequate rest at night. Your muscles recover faster when you sleep, because your body produces more muscle-building hormones when you're asleep. Aim to get seven to nine hours of sleep every night.

Nutrition What you eat also plays a major role in how quickly you recover. Your muscles need nutrients such as carbohydrates, proteins, fats, vitamins, and minerals to repair damaged muscles. If you find yourself struggling with recovery, take a look at your diet and make sure you are eating lots of whole, nutritious foods, especially in the hours after your workout.

By building in proper recovery, you can stay on track to become a better runner each week and avoid training too hard.

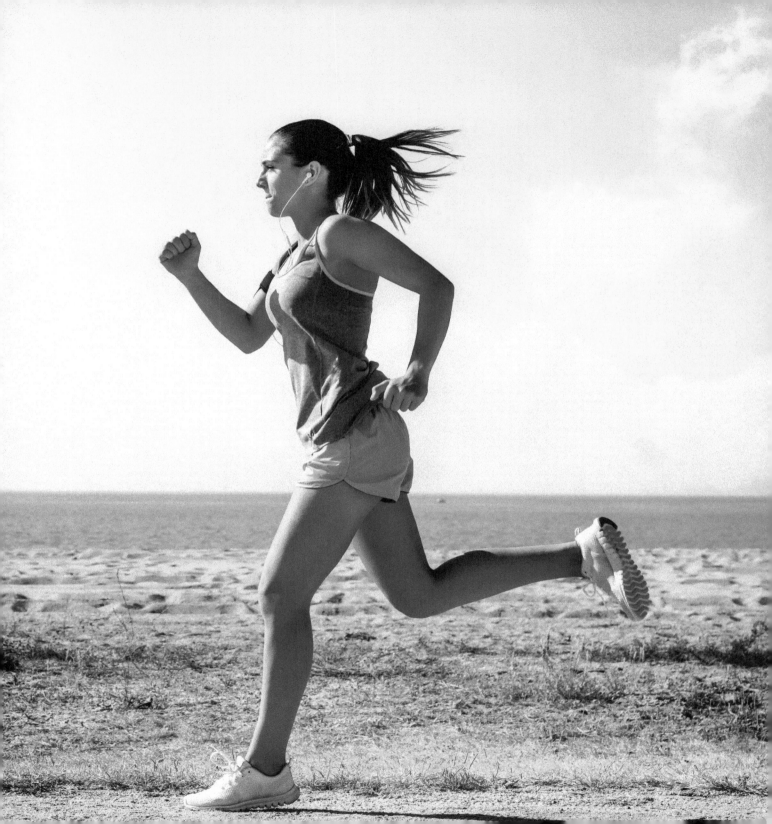

PART THREE

PUTTING IN THE WORK

In the previous chapters, I outlined the fundamentals of running and gave you the tools to stay injury-free as you train. In the following chapters, I'm going to put you to work with a series of drills and exercises that will help you solidify your technique, build strength, and execute your runs to the best of your ability. Let's do this!

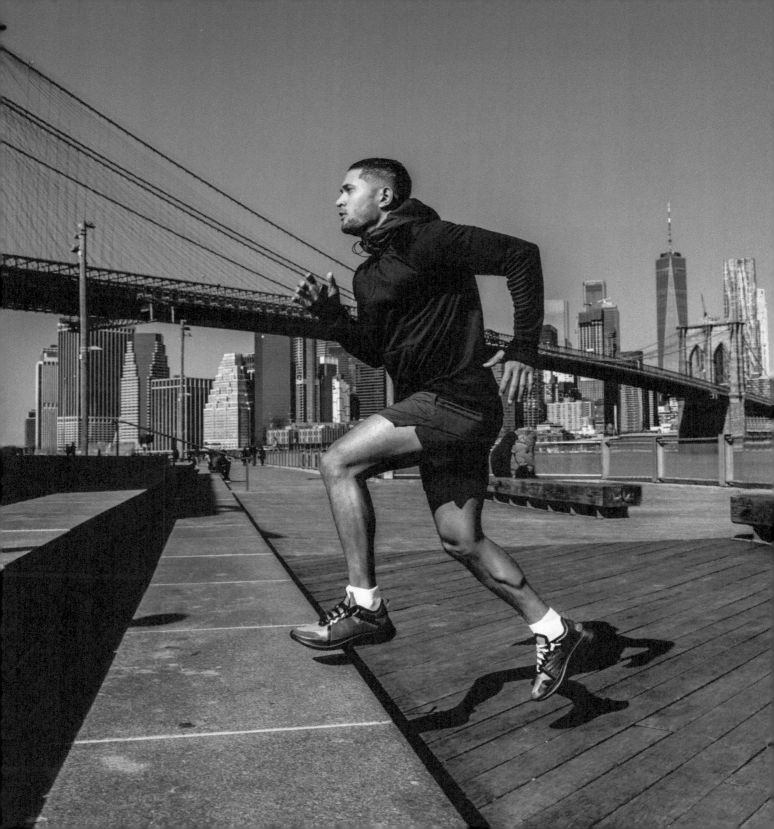

CHAPTER SIX

Technique Drills

In chapters 3 and 4, I discussed the mechanics of posture and alignment, as well as how to master your stride. Now that you understand the proper elements of good running form, it's time to implement technique drills to help you activate the right muscles and develop your strength.

What Are Technique Drills, Anyway?

In short, technique drills are quick exercises designed to hone the individual elements of proper running form. Just as a pianist's fingers move thoughtlessly across a keyboard to play a song he's practiced over and over again, these drills can help our bodies commit to memory the movements that are critical to a fundamentally sound run. Because an entire kinetic chain of events transpires with every step you take, you can't focus on, say, the way your hips move while you're actually running. But by breaking your overall form into isolated sections, you can effectively zero in on one element at a time.

These drills will strengthen the muscle groups needed for running—particularly muscles in the feet, calves, shins, glutes, and hips. And unlike traditional strength training exercises, these drills take your joints through a range of motion that is similar to that of running, strengthening the muscles in the exact manner in which they'll be used.

Drilling Down

Here are the primary aspects of your running form that technique drills will help improve—from the ground up.

Foot strike As you may recall from chapter 4, foot strike is where your foot first contacts the ground when you start the gait cycle. Technique drills help you develop a better awareness of your foot strike and shift, so your foot lands under your body, rather than in front of you.

Glute activation If you want to run fast and stay injury-free, you need to use your glutes to their maximum capacity. Due to poor posture and lots of sitting, many runners are unable to activate their glutes properly. Technique drills help recondition your body to fire these muscles.

Hip extension Hip extension is when you drive your upper thigh and leg backward after your foot makes contact with the ground. This component is perhaps the most critical one to generating a powerful stride.

Knee lift Knee lift is the degree to which you drive your leg forward during your running stride. Knee lift is connected to hip extension because the farther you lift your knee, the farther back your opposite leg can travel. Poor knee lift often causes overstriding.

Technique Terminology

Let's review some concepts commonly associated with technique drills.

Kinetic chain This term refers to the interrelated groups of joints and muscles that work together to produce your running stride. No single element of your running form works on its own. For example, changing the position of your foot strike affects your hip extension, knee lift, and stride length. It's helpful to be cognizant of the entire kinetic chain when you're working on your form.

Proprioception This is your body's internal sense of positioning and the motion of your joints and muscles when you move. With better awareness of your body's position as you run, you're more capable of moving with the proper stride. Research has also shown that increasing proprioception can reduce the likelihood of injuries (Myer et al. 2005).

Neuromuscular system This is the intricate communication system between your brain and your muscles. Improvements to the neuromuscular system allow your brain to send signals to your muscles faster so you can react more quickly and fire a greater percentage of muscle fibers with more force.

Flexion This term refers to your ability to move a joint or a part of your body closer together. In running, we primarily think of flexion in conjunction with the hip flexors, which enable you to bring your leg up toward your torso and bend your torso forward at the hip.

Extension This is the opposite of flexion, in that it refers to a movement that increases the angle or distance between body parts. Typically, we use this term in association with hip extension.

Ground contact time This is the amount of time your foot spends on the ground during the running stride. While ground contact time will always decrease as you run faster, it is possible to improve your contact time at all speeds, which helps you run with more power and, therefore, with greater speed.

Routines for Improving Your Technique

Implementing drills into your total-body running plan isn't complicated and doesn't require any special equipment. You can do these drills outside on a quiet street, at the track, or on an empty basketball or tennis court.

Technique drills also fit holistically into your running program and work in tandem with your running workouts, strength work, and other cross-training. The training plans in chapter 9 assign drill work on specific days. If you're building your own plan, include drills twice per week, on an easy day or a long run day. Always perform the drills after your run.

If you're a beginner or new to running drills, focus on performing each drill correctly and with proper form. It's better to do only half the repetitions or sets with good form than to rush through the routines with improper movements. If you're an experienced runner, you can reduce the drill sessions to once per week and choose the exercises that best target your weaknesses.

In this section, I'll describe the purpose and makeup of the two routines. In the next section, you'll find instructions on how to perform each drill.

Power Drill Routine (PD)

This routine focuses on developing proper movement patterns in the hips, glutes, hamstrings, and hip flexors. The routine should take only 10 to 15 minutes to complete. Remember, the goal of technique drills is to improve your mechanics, not to get in an aerobic workout, so don't hesitate to rest longer than suggested. If you're an experienced runner, you can perform an additional set for each drill to make the drills more challenging.

DRILL	REPS OR DISTANCE	SETS	REST
A-skips	20 steps total (10 each leg)	2	45 to 60 sec
B-skips	24 steps total (12 each leg)	2	60 to 90 sec
Straight Leg Bound	20 steps total (10 each leg)	1	60 to 90 sec
Butt Kicks	20 steps total (10 each leg)	2	30 to 45 sec
Carioca	8 crossovers, each direction	2	30 to 45 sec

Quick Feet Drill Routine (QR)

This routine focuses on improving ground contact time and lower leg awareness. The routine should take only 10 to 15 minutes to complete.

DRILL	REPS OR DISTANCE	SETS	REST
B-skips	24 steps total (12 each leg)	2	60 to 90 sec
Straight Leg Bound	20 steps total (10 each leg)	1	60 to 90 sec
Quick Feet	30 steps total (15 each leg)	2	60 to 90 sec
Ankling	20 steps total (10 each leg)	2	60 to 90 sec
High Knee	20 steps total (10 each leg)	2	30 to 45 sec

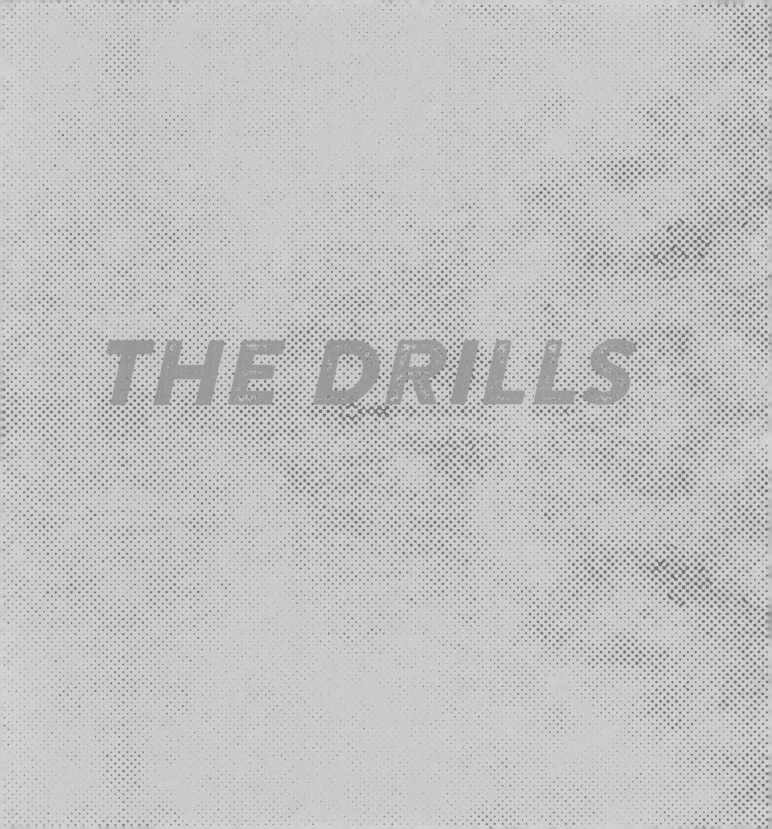

THE DRILLS

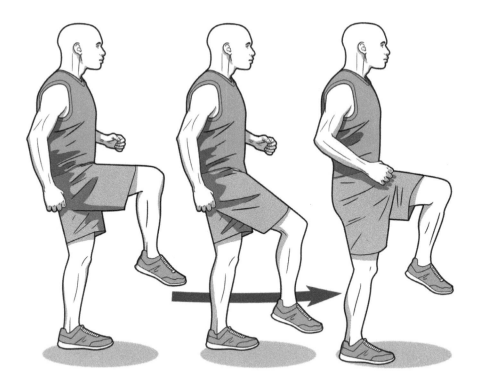

A-SKIPS

Areas worked: Foot strike and knee lift

1. Skip forward by using your ankle and foot muscles to lift yourself off the ground about two to three inches while moving forward about one foot.

2. While you skip, lift your lead knee as high as your waist and keep your back leg straight as you come off your toe.

3. Continue moving forward by skipping—alternating legs— and striking the ground with your midfoot or forefoot while swinging your opposite arm in unison with your lead leg.

BEGINNER TIP: When doing this drill for the first time, walk through it to get the motion down and gradually progress to skipping.

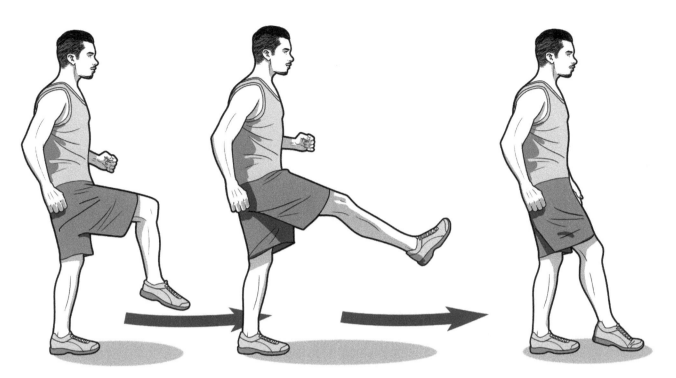

B-SKIPS

Areas worked: Glutes and hamstrings

1. Skip forward by using your ankle and foot muscles to lift yourself off the ground about two to three inches while moving forward about one foot. Exaggerate the lifting of your opposite leg.

2. Extend the leg you lifted off the ground. Slightly bending your leg is okay.

3. Rapidly accelerate the leg down by contracting or activating your hamstring muscle.

4. Repeat with your opposite leg in a skipping fashion.

BEGINNER TIP: When doing this drill for the first time, walk through it to get the motion down and gradually progress to skipping.

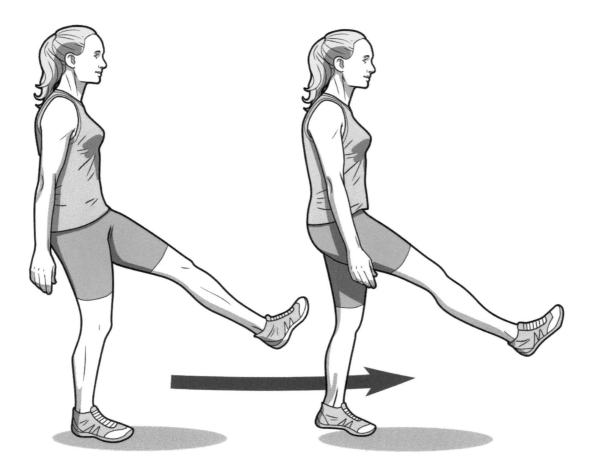

STRAIGHT LEG BOUND

Areas worked: Glutes and hamstrings

1. Keeping your legs straight, use your hamstring and glute to move yourself forward on one leg. Land on the ball of your foot of the opposite leg.

2. Keeping both legs straight, again, repeat the motion by using your hamstring and glute to propel yourself forward. It should feel like you're trying to run but without bending at the knees.

BEGINNER TIP: If you'd like to see a video demonstration of this drill, you can find a link in the Resources appendix (see page 151).

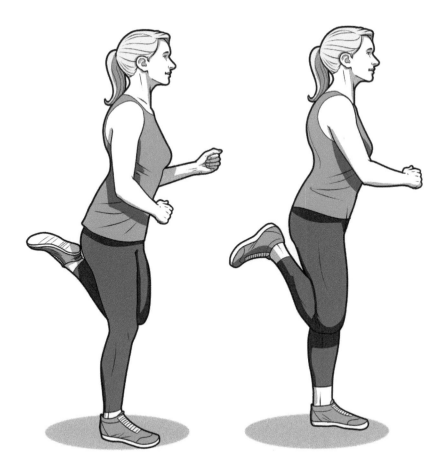

BUTT KICKS

Areas worked: Leg turnover and recovery

1. Keeping your thighs in a locked position, run in place.

2. Try to kick yourself in the buttocks with your heel on each stride.

BEGINNER TIP: Focus on keeping the rest of your body still and simply flicking your lower leg backward.

CARIOCA

Areas worked: Glute and hip mobility

1. Standing upright with your head and torso facing forward, move laterally in one direction by placing your trailing leg in front of your lead leg.

2. Shift back to a neutral position.

3. Move the lead leg in that same lateral direction and place the trailing leg in front of the lead leg.

4. Continue in the same motion, repeating from step 1.

5. Complete eight steps in one direction. Then reverse direction and swap legs, performing the same movement.

BEGINNER TIP: If you'd like to see a video demonstration of this drill, you can find a link in the Resources appendix (see page 151).

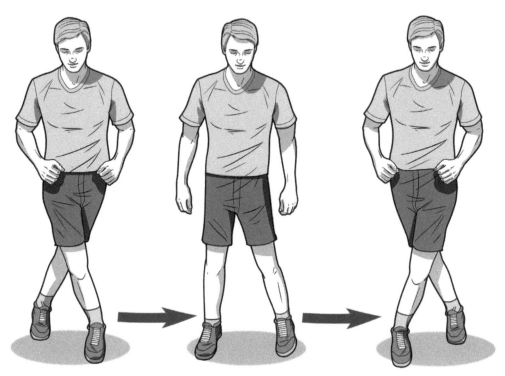

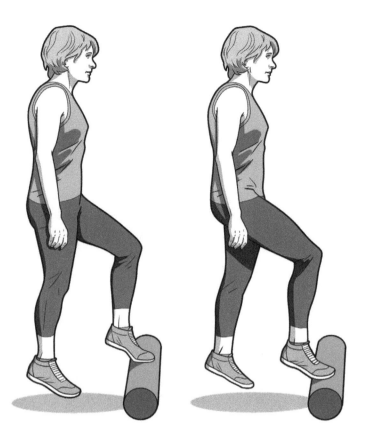

QUICK FEET

Area worked: Ground contact time

1. Standing with a slight forward lean at the ankle, place a small object in front of you that is no more than two feet high, such as a shoe box or a basketball.

2. Move your feet up and down, tapping your forefoot on the object.

3. Start slow and increase the speed/cadence as you get more comfortable.

BEGINNER TIP: Good household options are a step stool, small box, basketball, or even a roadside curb.

ANKLING

Areas worked: Ankle strength and ground contact time

1. Start with both feet on the ground, knees slightly bent.

2. Lift your right heel while keeping your toes on the ground. Try to initiate the movement from your ankle by pressing down on your toes, not just lifting your heel up.

3. Rapidly thrust your right heel down toward the ground. At the same time, scoot your left foot forward about three inches and use your ankle to raise your left heel off the ground.

4. Without stopping, thrust your left heel back toward the ground while scooting forward with your right foot by raising your heel off the ground.

5. Continue to repeat this movement.

BEGINNER TIP: If you'd like to see a video demonstration of this drill, you can find a link in the Resources appendix (see page 151).

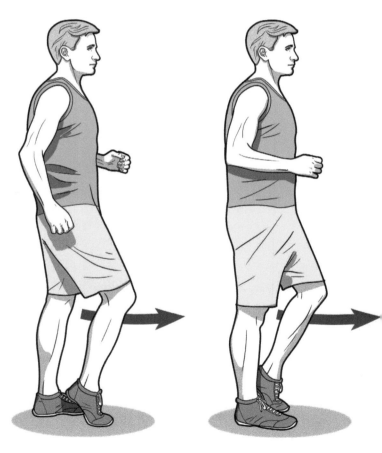

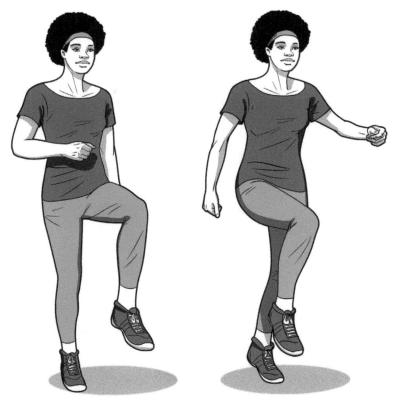

HIGH KNEE

Areas worked: Glutes, hamstring power, and knee lift

1. With very quick cadence, thrust your left knee upward until your thigh breaks a plane parallel to the ground.

2. Bring the leg back down, focusing on soft, flat foot strikes near the ball of your foot.

3. As soon as the first foot hits the ground, repeat with your other leg. You should essentially be running in place, using this form.

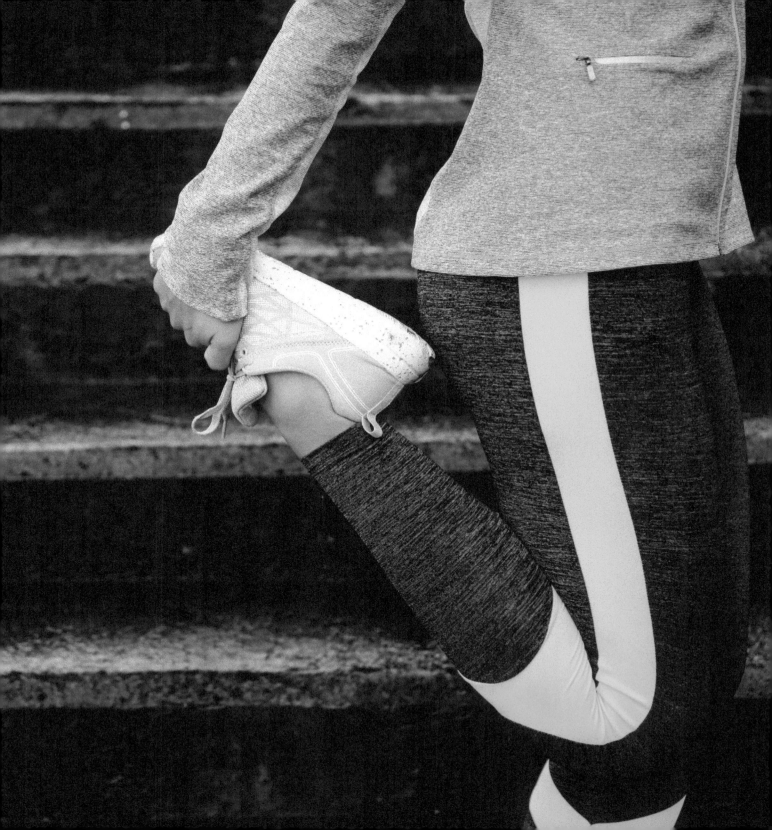

CHAPTER SEVEN

Strength Workouts

The key to long-term progress, staying injury-free, and continual improvement as a runner is strengthening your entire body. You can't just focus on adding more miles or doing faster workouts and expect to improve. When you integrate strength training into your running plan, you become a more powerful runner.

One common misconception about strength training is that you need expensive equipment for your workout to be productive. But while you should feel free to hit the gym or incorporate free weight and barbell exercises into your workouts, research shows that body-weight strength training alone is effective for building running strength and reducing your risk of injury (Ferruati et al. 2010).

In this chapter, I've created five simple bodyweight strength routines, expressly designed to make you a stronger runner. All of them will be integrated into the training schedules in chapter 9.

Equipment

All the exercises in this chapter can be performed without any equipment. However, as you get stronger, you may want to increase the difficulty. To do this, you can incorporate the following pieces of equipment:

- Kettlebells
- Resistance bands
- Dumbbells
- Household items, such as an empty milk jug

Use the kettlebells, dumbbells, and milk jug (filled with water to desired heaviness) to add resistance to exercises such as the lunge and squat. In the exercises that involve pulling (arms or legs), you can use resistance bands to increase the difficulty.

A Brief Introduction to Cross-Training

Cross-training is useful for improving your aerobic endurance without putting pressure on your legs. Unfortunately, most runners don't implement cross-training until they are already injured. Adding regular cross-training to your schedule can help you become a stronger, faster runner.

These are some of the best methods:

Aqua jogging This is a form of underwater running (your feet don't touch the bottom) that closely mimics the movements of actual jogging. It's the most effective method for building and maintaining your running body.

Biking Although pedaling doesn't simulate the running motion, biking does enable you to increase your heart rate and work your quads in a way that is similar to running hills. Biking is a good option if you want a harder workout.

Elliptical Research shows that the elliptical can produce metabolic and cardiorespiratory improvements similar to those produced by running. The main difference between the two exercises is that the quads are activated more during elliptical training and impact rates are zero.

Swimming Swimming is a great cross-training method for breaking up the monotony of training. While swimming relies primarily on the upper body for power, it efficiently challenges both aerobic endurance and VO_2 max (see page 105). Because swimming challenges different systems, it can be a great change of pace for runners looking to become better all-around athletes.

The Workouts

In this section, I'll describe the purpose of the strength workouts, each of which focuses on a different objective. The exercises included are proven to be the most effective for runners; instructions for how to perform them are at the end of this chapter. Each routine will take less than 20 minutes to complete.

If you're not following one of the sample training plans in chapter 9, incorporate leg strength or plyometric work into your harder running days, not on your easy or rest days. Core, hip, and general strength workouts are best performed on easy days or rest days.

Core

This routine helps you establish the foundation for a rock-solid core. The exercises aim to improve your running economy and maintain proper form, both of which contribute to faster times, stronger finishes, and less potential for injuries. The benefits are the result of targeting the core in all planes of motion, focusing on all-around power, springiness, and mobility.

Core Routine (CR)

EXERCISE	REPETITIONS	SETS	REST
Plank	Hold for 30 to 45 sec	2	60 sec
Bicycle	15 rotations each direction	2	60 sec
Mountain Climbers	10 each leg	2	90 sec
Bracers	Hold for 60 sec	2	30 sec
Reach Out and Back	10 each leg	2	90 sec

Lower Body

This routine dynamically targets the quads, hips, and glutes to develop running-specific strength to solidify proper form, build resistance to injuries, and create more explosiveness through your stride.

Lower-Body Routine (LB)

EXERCISE	REPETITIONS	SETS	REST
Pistol Squat	5 each leg	3	90 sec
Lunge	10 each leg	2	60 sec
Calf Raises	15	2	45 sec
Water Pump	10 each leg	3	90 sec

General Strength

This routine is designed to help you become a more well-rounded athlete. Performing general upper-body strength exercises can help prevent injury and ensure you maintain good form late in the race.

General Strength Routine (GS)

EXERCISE	REPETITIONS	SETS	REST
Push-up	10	2	90 sec
Plank Row	15 each arm	2	60 sec
Shoulder Rotation	15	2	30 sec

Plyometrics

This routine combines multiple plyometric movements to develop power, improve running mechanics, and enhance rhythm, coordination, and strength to prevent injuries.

Plyometrics Routine (PL)

EXERCISE	REPETITIONS	SETS	REST
Squat Jump	10	3	90 sec
Water Pump	10 each leg	3	90 sec
Skips for Height	10 each leg	2	90 sec
Ankle Jumps	20	3	60 sec

Hips and Glutes

Numerous scientific studies have proven that runners routinely suffer from weak, tight, and underdeveloped hip muscles (Fredericson et al. 2010; Ireland et al. 2003; Niemuth et al. 2005). A strength workout that doubles as an injury-prevention routine, this set of exercises works all the muscles in the hips and glutes, while also increasing flexibility and range of motion.

The Art (and Science) of Plyometrics

Plyometrics are explosive jumping exercises that use the stretch-shortening concept to help develop power and improve running efficiency.

The stretch-shortening concept refers to how your muscles, tendons, and ligaments store energy as you bend them and then release that energy when they're extended. This principle is why, for example, you can jump higher if you bend at the knees. The goal of plyometrics is to improve your ability to store energy and release it so your muscles can do more work using less energy.

Research has shown just how effective plyometric exercises can be. One study on well-trained endurance athletes found that adding plyometrics to their normal training plans improved their 5k race times (Paavolainen et al. 1999). Another study found that plyometrics improved participants' overall running economy by 2.3 percent (Turner et al. 2003).

The downside to plyometrics is that the exercises are difficult on the body. You'll only want to do this workout once a week, and taper them off the closer you get to a race day.

Hips and Glutes Routine (HP)

EXERCISE	REPETITIONS	SETS	REST
Bridge	Hold 30 sec	3	60 sec
Bird Dog	12 each side	2	60 sec
Hip Extension	15 each leg	3	60 sec
Clamshell	15 each side	3	60 sec

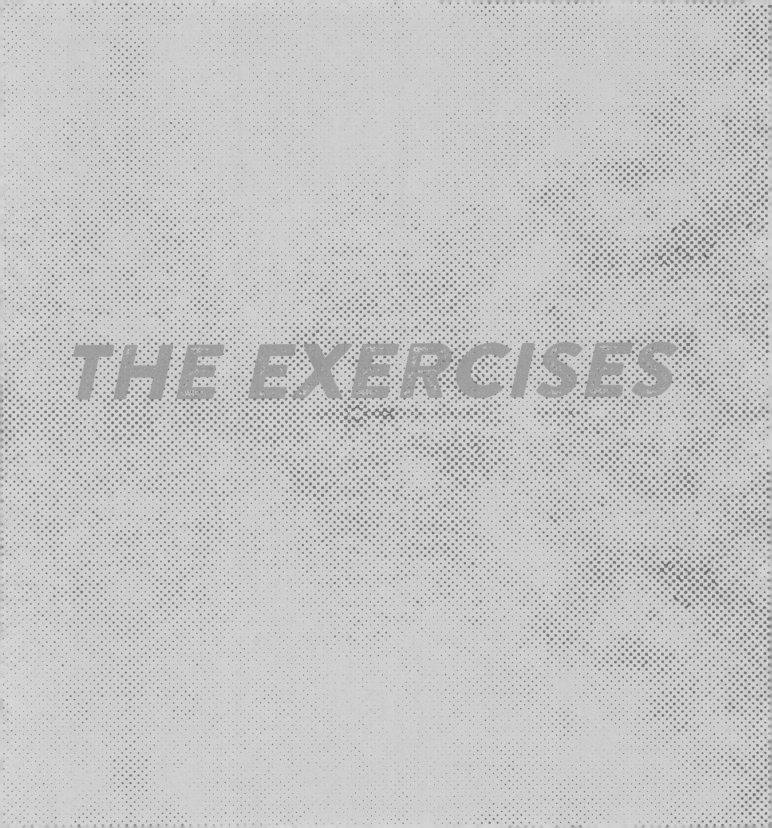

THE EXERCISES

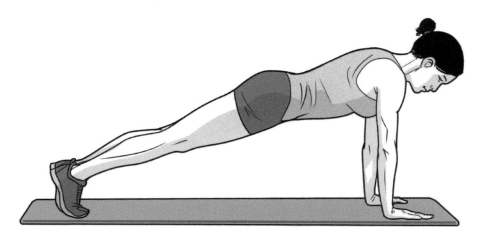

PLANK

Area worked: Core

1. Plant your hands under your shoulders (slightly wider than shoulder width) like you're about to do a push-up.

2. Ground your toes into the floor and squeeze your glutes to stabilize your body.

3. Neutralize your neck and spine by looking at a spot on the floor about a foot beyond your hands. Your head should be in line with your back.

4. Brace your core (tighten your abs) and hold this position.

LEVEL UP: To make this exercise more difficult, rest on your elbows and forearms instead of your hands.

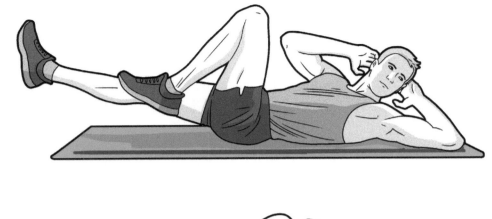

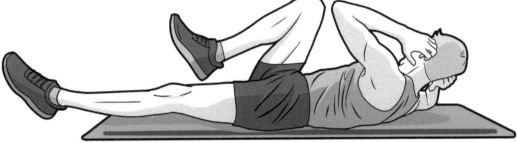

BICYCLE

Area worked: Obliques

1. Lie flat on your back with your core braced and your hands behind your head.

2. Bring your right leg toward your chest while lifting your head and twisting to touch your left elbow to your knee.

3. Bring your leg back down and repeat with the opposite arm and leg.

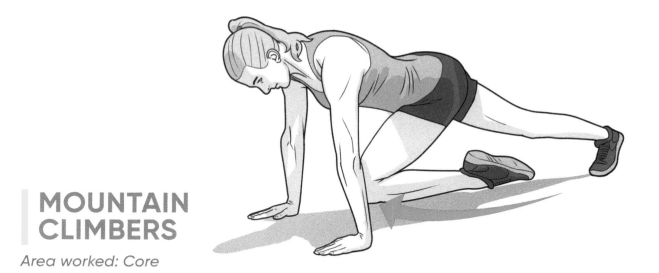

MOUNTAIN CLIMBERS

Area worked: Core

1. Begin on your hands and knees. Your heels should be up and your toes should be pointed toward the floor.

2. Move your left foot forward and place it on the floor under your chest. Your knee and hip should be bent and your thigh should be in toward your chest.

3. Lift your right knee up off the floor, making your right leg straight and strong. Your right toes should be tucked beneath you, heel up. Brace your core to stabilize your spine.

4. Keeping your hands firmly on the floor and your core engaged and shoulders strong, jump to switch leg positions. Both feet should leave the ground as you drive your right knee forward and reach your left leg back. At this point, your left leg is fully extended behind you and your right knee and hip are bent with your right foot on the floor.

5. Repeat as fast as you can with good control.

BRACERS

Areas worked: Hip flexors and core

1. Lie on your back with your knees bent at a 90-degree angle and your shins lifted and parallel to the floor.

2. Place your right hand on your right knee and your left hand on your left knee.

3. Brace your core and press your hands as hard as possible into your knees, while your knees resist the pressure from your hands. Aim to keep your lower back on the floor.

4. Hold this position for the duration of the exercise time.

LEVEL UP: Maximize gains by pressing your lower back onto the floor while contracting your stomach.

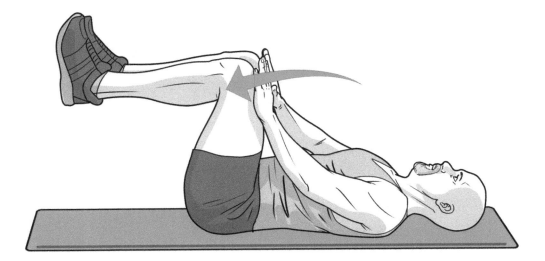

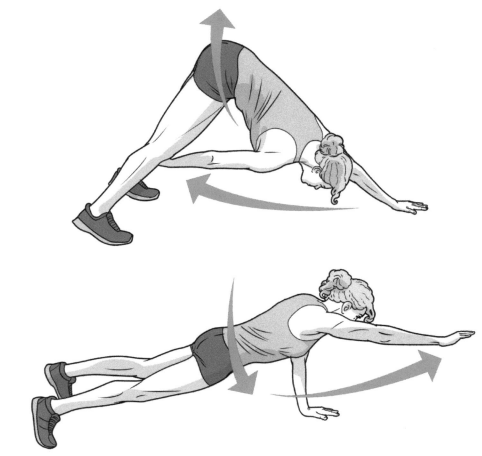

REACH OUT AND BACK

Areas worked: Core and shoulders

1. Set up in a plank position on your hands and toes—shoulders over your wrists and feet hip-distance apart.

2. Push your hips in the air as you reach your right hand back toward your left ankle.

3. Return to the high plank position by extending your hips and simultaneously reaching your right hand out in front of you. Then perform the same movement.

BEGINNER TIP: Don't let your hips sag as you reach forward. Focus on engaging your glutes and keeping your core super tight.

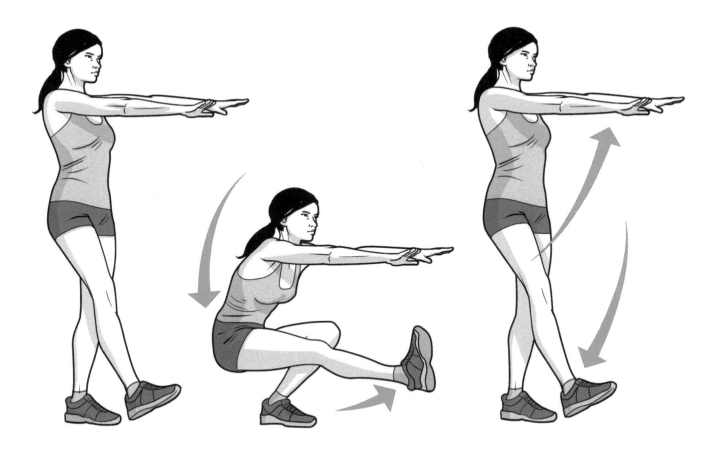

PISTOL SQUAT

Areas worked: Core, hamstrings, and quads

1. Start by standing on one leg, with your toes pointed forward or slightly turned out.

2. Slowly sit down into a squat, making sure that your torso leans slightly forward (similar to a back squat).

3. Once you have assumed a deep squat position, use your single leg strength to press into the floor, locking your core tight for maximal effort.

LUNGE

Areas worked: Hamstrings and quads

1. Stand tall with feet hip-width apart. Engage your core.

2. Take a big step forward with your right leg and start to shift your weight forward so the heel of your right foot hits the floor first.

3. Lower your body until your right thigh is parallel to the floor and your right shin is vertical. It's okay if your knee shifts forward a little, as long as it doesn't go past your right toe. If mobility allows, lightly tap your left knee to the ground, while keeping your weight on the right heel.

4. Press into your right heel to drive back up to the starting position.

5. Repeat on the other side.

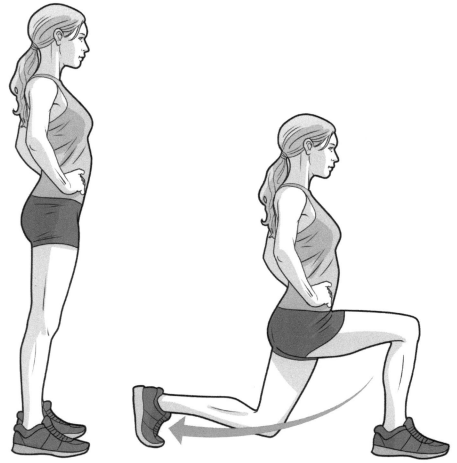

CALF RAISES

Area worked: Calves

1. From a standing position, slowly rise on your toes, keeping your knees straight and heels off the floor.

2. Hold briefly, then come back down.

LEVEL UP: Try standing on something elevated (such as a stairstep) to achieve a wider range of motion.

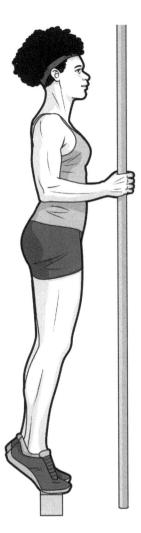
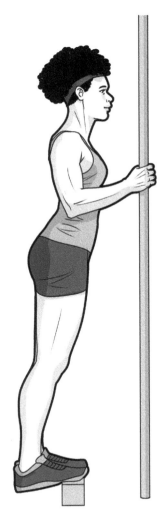

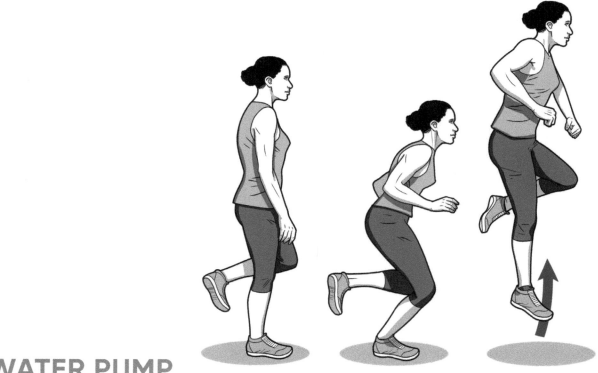

WATER PUMP

Areas worked: Calves and quads

1. Place your left foot about three to four feet behind your body.

2. Slowly bend down on your right leg until you are a few degrees from being parallel.

3. Explode up and jump into the air.

4. Land on your right foot.

5. Rest one to three seconds and repeat for the recommended repetitions. Once finished, repeat using the opposite leg.

BEGINNER TIP: In step 1, feel free to rest your foot on a chair or an object of a similar height.

PUSH-UP

Areas worked: Shoulders and triceps

1. Start in a high plank position. Place your hands firmly on the ground, directly under your shoulders. Ground your toes into the floor to stabilize your lower half.

2. Begin to lower your body—keeping your back flat and eyes focused about three feet in front of you to maintain a neutral neck—until your chest grazes the floor. Your body should remain in a straight line from head to toe.

3. Draw your shoulder blades back and down, keeping your elbows tucked close to your body. (Don't let your elbows flare out to a T position.)

4. Keeping your core engaged, exhale as you push back to the starting position.

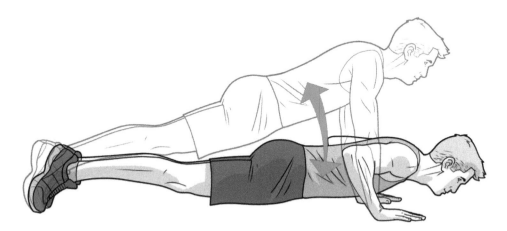

PLANK ROW

Areas worked: Back, core, and shoulders

1. Start on your hands and toes, hip-width distance apart, in a standard plank position.

2. Bend your right elbow and slowly lift it up toward the ceiling, keeping your elbow in tight by your side.

3. Lower the arm and repeat on the other side.

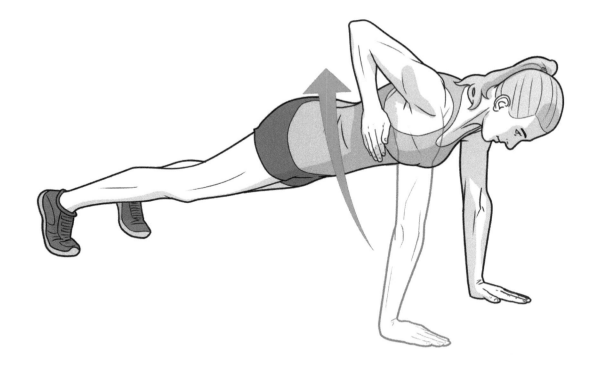

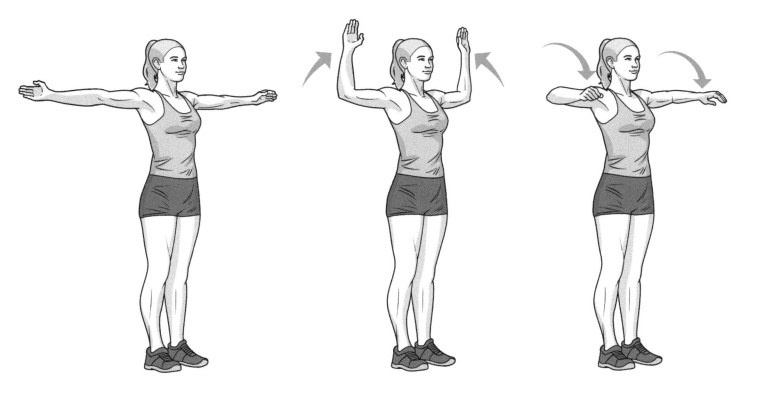

SHOULDER ROTATION

Area worked: Rotator cuffs

1. Begin with your arms straight out by your side.

2. Bend your elbows so your arms form an L shape.

3. Keeping the same bend in your arm, slowly rotate your shoulders forward until your arms are parallel with the ground.

4. Hold for one second and then raise your arms back up.

LEVEL UP: Hold a small weight in each hand to increase the difficulty.

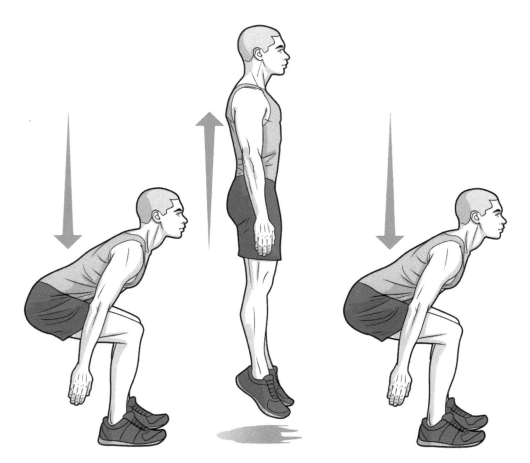

SQUAT JUMP

Areas worked: Calves, glutes, hamstrings, and quads

1. Stand with your feet shoulder-width apart.

2. Start by doing a regular squat—slowly lower yourself by bending at the knees and hips.

3. Once your legs are parallel to the floor, engage your core and jump up explosively.

LEVEL UP: When you land, lower your body back into the squat position to complete one repetition. Try to land as softly as possible, which requires greater control.

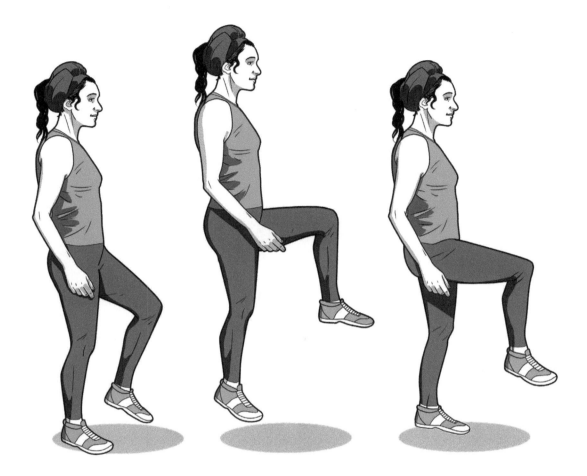

SKIPS FOR HEIGHT

Area worked: Improves power

1. Skip as high as you can, raising your knee as high as possible while forcefully extending your drive up.

2. Land, then repeat using the alternate leg. Continue to cycle back and forth between legs.

BEGINNER TIP: The key is to get as much height as possible, so explode off the ground into each skip as fast as possible.

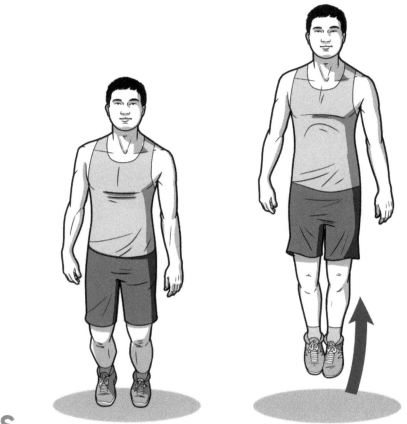

ANKLE JUMPS

Areas worked: Ankle and foot strength

1. Stand with your feet close together and your knees slightly bent.

2. Using only your ankles, thrust yourself into the air. Try not to bend your legs.

3. Land on your forefeet, pause for two seconds, and repeat.

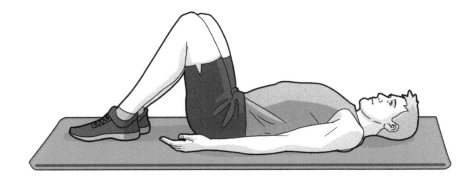

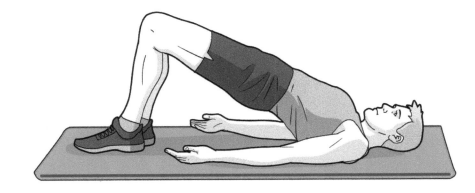

BRIDGE

Areas worked: Glutes and hips

1. Lie on your back with your knees bent and core engaged.

2. Keeping your shoulder blades on the ground, engage your glutes and hips to slowly raise your buttocks off the ground.

3. Your body should form a straight line at the top of the movement. Hold for 30 seconds. Don't let your hips sag.

4. Slowly lower back down.

LEVEL UP: To increase the difficulty, hold a weight on your pelvis or perform the exercise with one leg at a time, keeping the non-working leg straight and parallel with the working leg.

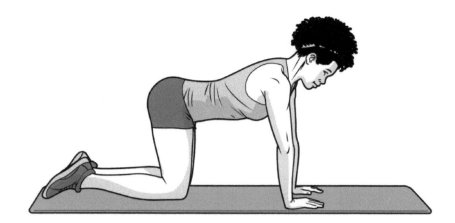

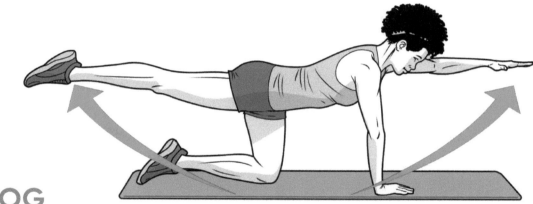

BIRD DOG

Area worked: Core

1. Start on your hands and knees, keeping your shoulders over your wrists and your hips over your knees.

2. Engaging your abs, reach your left arm forward so it is in line with your ear. At the same time, extend your right leg straight back.

3. Return to the starting position and repeat on the other side.

LEVEL UP: To increase the difficulty, begin in the plank position on your palms and toes rather than your knees.

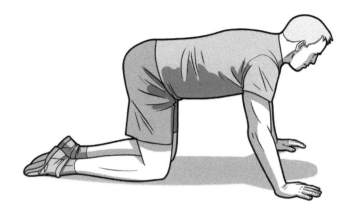

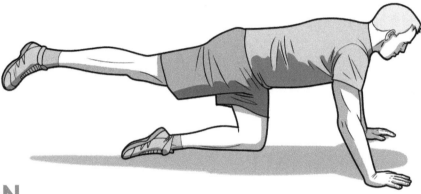

HIP EXTENSION

Areas worked: Glutes and hips

1. Begin on your hands and knees. Keep your abs tight and your back flat.

2. Slowly lift one leg backward, using your glute to initiate the movement.

3. Return your leg so you're back on your hands and knees. Repeat with the other leg.

LEVEL UP: Wrap a resistance band around the knee that's on the ground and your opposite foot to create tension and make this exercise more difficult.

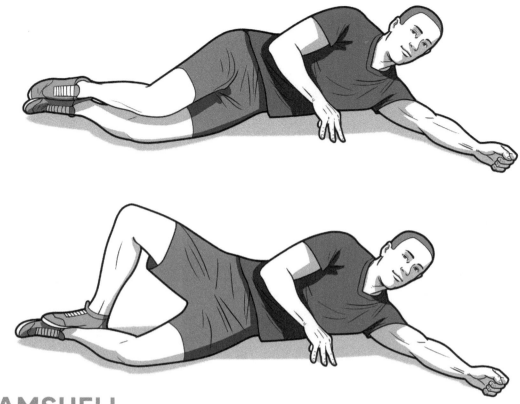

CLAMSHELL

Area worked: Hips

1. Lie on your side with both legs bent.

2. Keeping your feet together and your pelvis perpendicular to the floor, lift the top knee into the air.

3. Hold at the top for two to three seconds.

4. Return to the starting position. Once you've finished all repetitions on one side, turn over and repeat with the opposite hip and leg.

LEVEL UP: Wrap a resistance band around your knees to create tension and make this exercise more difficult.

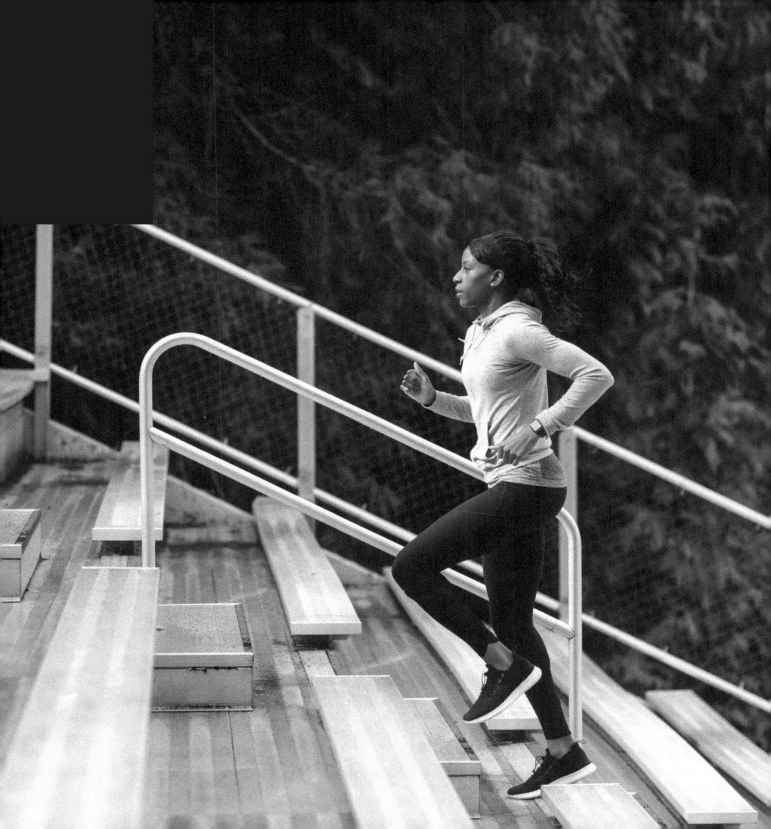

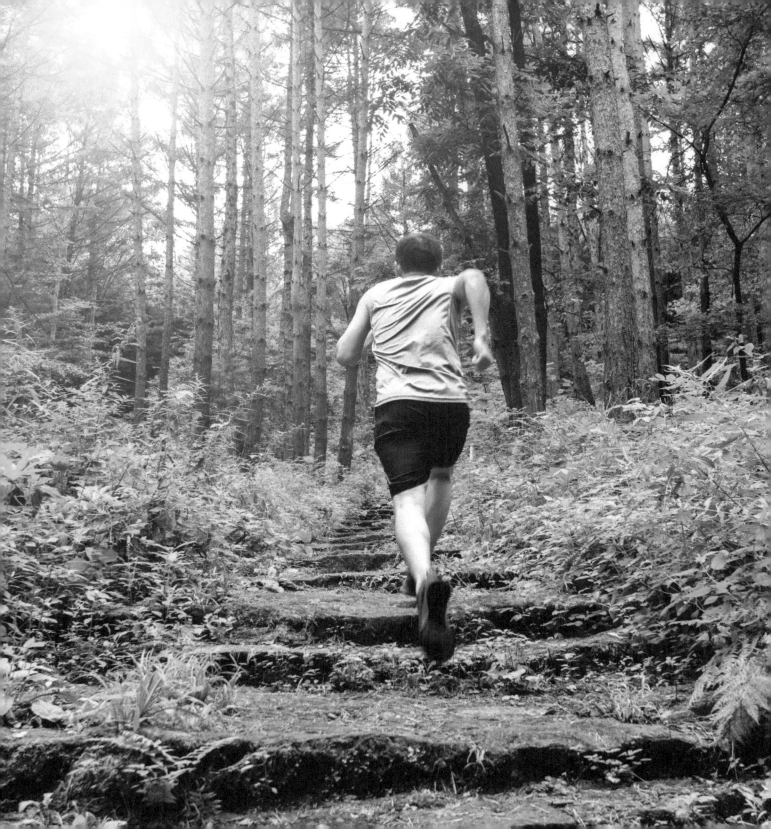

CHAPTER EIGHT

Types of Runs

Simply running as hard or as far as you can each day is not the ideal way to train. In fact, doing so will forestall your progress. To continually improve (and stay injury-free), you need to incorporate different types of runs into your training. Each type of run outlined in this chapter has a particular purpose and elicits a specific change or improvement to your fitness.

Establishing Pace

The fundamental difference between different types of runs is the pace. If you don't run at the correct pace, then you're not going to get the intended benefit of the workout.

Knowing how to effectively pace yourself during a race is one of the most integral skills you can develop. To achieve your fastest time on race day, you need to become a pacing pro who can feel the difference between just a few seconds' variance in your pace. Research has shown that runners who start a 5k race just a few seconds too fast, for example, run 10 percent slower and have a 6 percent greater chance of not finishing (Gosztyla et al. 2006).

How to Keep Pace

There are no shortcuts to improving your pacing—it simply requires practice. But here are three strategies to bear in mind:

Stop relying on your watch Run-tracking apps and watches are great tools, but you don't want to get into the habit of checking your watch every 10 to 15 seconds. Instead, glance at your watch during the first few minutes of your run to make sure you're on pace, and don't look at it again until you've finished.

Monitor your breathing Being aware of your breath is integral to identifying your pace. When you land on the right pace for a run or workout, you'll notice a shift in your breathing rhythm if you happen to speed up or slow down.

Use the track It's much easier to control your pace without hills or stoplights slowing you up. Running on a track will give you constant and accurate feedback, which will help you begin to feel slight pace variations.

The Six Essential Runs

We've covered the fundamentals and workouts. Now it's time to run. The following overview covers the most important runs.

Intervals

An interval is any running workout where you split the distance into shorter sections with rest in between. When running intervals, you can change the purpose of the run by manipulating three variables—the length of the interval, the amount of rest, and the pace you run. Generally speaking, intervals can be grouped into two categories: VO_2 max, or anaerobic, intervals and threshold, or cruise, intervals.

VO_2 Max or Anaerobic Intervals

These intervals are shorter—typically no longer than 1,000 meters—run at or near your fastest pace possible, and include long rest times, usually equal to the amount of time you spend running. These types of workouts are primarily for shorter races, such as the 5k and 10k.

What Exactly Is VO₂ Max?

VO$_2$ max is a measure of the maximum volume of oxygen your body can process when you are running. The faster your body can process oxygen, the faster you'll be able to run without having to take a breather. With this pace, you are requiring your body to process as much oxygen as fast as it can. The long rest ensures you're not producing too much lactate—a substance produced in your body when you burn glycogen—for your body to process.

Threshold or Cruise Interval

These intervals are usually longer—800 meters to a mile—run at or just faster than your threshold pace, and include short rest periods. Threshold intervals allow you to run much faster than a tempo run (see below), but because of the short rest, you can maintain a threshold effort. These types of workouts are primarily for runners racing the half marathon and marathon.

While your threshold pace varies depending on how much you train, it should feel like a hard but controlled effort, typically featuring a two-to-two breathing rhythm (see page 106).

Tempo Runs

Tempo runs are designed to train your body to run at the aforementioned pace, otherwise known as your *lactate threshold*—the point at which you start to generate more lactic acid than your body can convert back into energy. Ultimately, the more efficient your body becomes at clearing lactate, the faster you can run without your muscles starting to fail.

Tempo runs are critical for every runner, whether you're training for a race or just trying to get in better shape. There are a few kinds of tempo runs you can include in your running plan.

Short Tempo

Short tempo runs are two to four miles, but they are executed at a slightly faster pace— typically near the upper limit of your threshold. These runs help your body learn to clear out lactate more efficiently. Short tempo runs are more important for 5k and 10k runners. During these runs, your breathing should be harder but controlled.

Long Tempo

Longer tempo runs can be three to eight miles long and are executed at a slightly slower pace—usually on the lower end of your lactate threshold. As you become more tired, running at the same pace becomes increasingly more difficult. Longer tempo runs teach your body how to clear lactate as you get fatigued. These runs are critical for runners who race half and full marathons. During these runs, your breathing should be controlled but not easy.

Tempo Intervals

It's difficult, especially for beginners, to run two, three, or five miles at threshold pace. To make it easier for all runners (even experienced ones) to run longer at lactate threshold pace, tempo runs can be broken into sections, with a short rest to help lower your lactate levels. For example, you could complete two runs, each two miles long, at your lactate threshold pace. Tempo intervals are useful for maintaining fitness and for runners who are training for any distance. During these runs, your breathing should be harder but controlled.

Take a Deep Breath . . .

Naturally, breathing is an important part of running, and, believe it or not, there's a right way and a wrong way to do it.

First, you should always breathe through your mouth when running. Initiate your breathing from your diaphragm (the top of your belly), not your chest. As you breathe, your stomach should expand and contract as your diaphragm forces air in and out of your lungs. Your chest, meanwhile, should remain mostly still.

If you're having difficulty breathing or you're quickly running out of breath when you run, pay attention to your *breathing rhythm*. Breathing rhythm refers to the number of steps you take with each foot while breathing in or out. For example, a two-to-two rhythm means you take two steps (one with your right foot and one with you left) while breathing in, and two steps while breathing out. Your exact breathing rhythm will depend on how hard you are running.

Typically, a three-to-three rhythm (three steps—one with your left, one with your right, one with your left—while breathing in, and three steps while breathing out) works best for warm-ups and most easy runs. Harder runs should typically be performed at a two-to-two rhythm. At the end of races or during the final push of a particularly hard interval session, you can switch to a one-to-two or two-to-one breathing rhythm.

Hill Repeats

Hill repeats are a type of interval session where you run up a hill as fast as you can and walk back down it for rest. These runs are perfect for boosting your VO_2 max and increasing muscle strength. The powerful contractions from the lifting of the hips, glutes, and quads up the hill share the same basic mechanics as plyometrics (see page 80). In essence, you get a lung-blasting running workout and a strength workout all in one.

Hill repeats are useful to all runners at different times in the training cycle. For shorter distance races, such as the 5k and 10k, as well as for general fitness, you can include hill repeats anytime. For longer races, such as the half and full marathon, it's best to complete hill repeats only in the beginning of your training cycle.

Long Runs

Many runners think long runs are only useful for the half and full marathon, but these runs are critical even for the 5k distance.

The length of a long run is the only factor that determines how it is implemented in a training plan. Essentially, you want to run the entire race distance at an easy pace, although you can make improvements with slightly shorter long runs.

Easy Runs

The number one mistake runners make is running their easy days too fast. It may seem that the faster you could do your easy runs, the quicker you would see results. But this reasoning couldn't be further from the truth.

An easy running day serves two purposes: to help you recover from your harder workouts and to improve your aerobic system. (The aerobic system refers to the process of breaking down and using energy during exercise when you have sufficient oxygen. For example, 99 percent of the energy for a half marathon and marathon will come from your aerobic system, compared to 95 percent for a 5k.)

The faster you run, the more you weaken your body's ability to recover, which increases your risk of injury and burnout. Additionally, research shows that running faster than about 65 percent of your 5k pace actually reduces the gains to your aerobic system (Dudley et al. 1982).

When your plan calls for an easy run, your pace should be easy enough that you could have a full conversation with someone beside you. Your run should not feel hard at all. Enjoy your run and remember: When it comes to easy runs, faster is not better!

Pace Training

At its core, training is about adaptation. Your body adapts to the demands you place on it by growing stronger and becoming more efficient. Although any kind of running improves your overall fitness, the best way to set a personal best at a specific race distance is to train at the pace you need for the race.

At the start of your training, you obviously won't be able to run at your race pace for the entire run. Therefore, you need to break up the distance and include short rest periods to recover.

Here's an example: A runner training for a 5k run might run 400 meters at race pace 10 times with 30-second rests in between (typically formatted as "10 x 400m with 30-second rest"). A 10k runner might do longer intervals, such as running 1,000 meters five times with 60-second rests in between. As you make progress, either the interval that you run at race pace should get longer or the amount of rest time between intervals should get shorter.

These types of runs are essential if you're planning to race any distance. If you're not planning to race, you don't need to include this type of run in your plan.

PART FOUR

TIME TO TRAIN

Now that you understand the physiology and philosophy behind a total-body running plan, you can put together a training schedule that will help you achieve your goals. Are you ready?

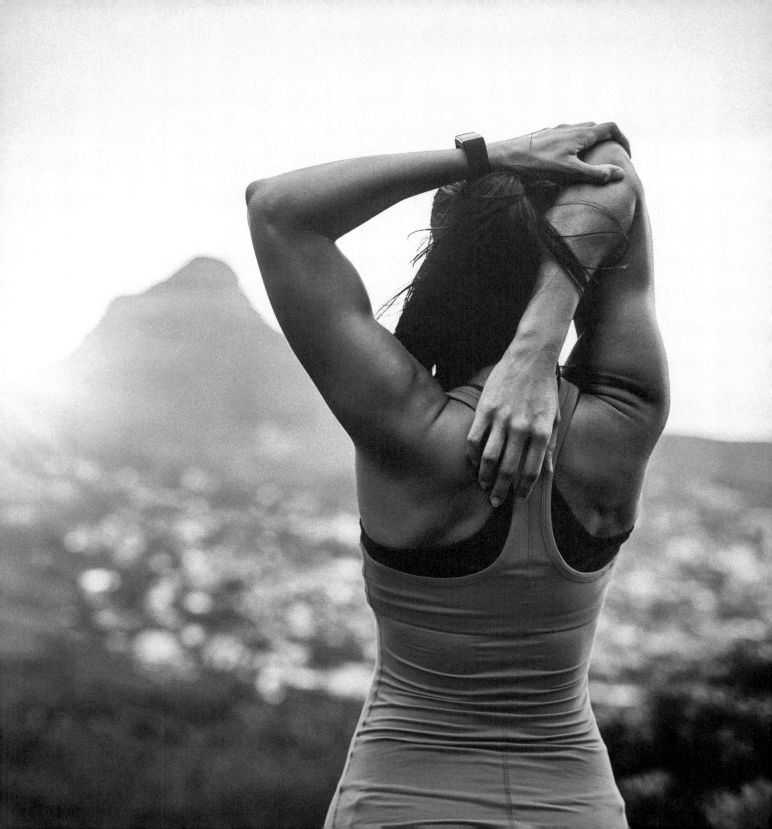

CHAPTER NINE

Your Total-Body Running Plan

Ready to run? Whether you simply want to become a stronger runner or you have a race distance in mind, these training plans provide an easy blueprint for you to follow.

The best way to execute these running plans is to first complete the run for the day, then perform any assigned stretching routine, and finish with strength training (of course, you should always do some warm-up stretches as well). This order allows you to focus on your running workout, ensures you eliminate any tightness with stretching, and leaves you with enough energy to complete your strength training.

The plans are designed to help you make consistent progress each week, so that by the end of the schedule, you're in peak running shape. All the plans include a combination of the routines covered in the previous chapters to ensure you stay healthy and maintain a strong foundation.

Still, no plan is one-size-fits-all. If you need to modify some of the workout days, or you would like to develop your own plan, refer to the principles in the Introduction to adjust the schedules as needed.

Sample Training Plans

I've provided seven different training plans along with some guidelines to help you choose the one that's right for you.

New Runners (see page 113): This 10-week plan is for those who have not run much before, or who have been running consistently for three to six months. The schedule starts off very easy and does not include any speed or tempo workouts.

Noncompetitive Novices (see page 118): Novices are still new to running but have been training on their own for about six months and are ready to follow a more structured plan. Ideally, when you choose this eight-week plan, you'll already be comfortable running three times per week and averaging about 10 to 15 miles per week.

Noncompetitive Intermediate Runners (see page 122): Intermediate runners have between six months to a year of running experience. Ideally, when you choose this eight-week plan, you'll already be comfortable running 15 to 20 miles per week.

Running Your First 5k (see page 126): This 12-week plan is designed for those who have been running for at least six months and wish to compete in their first 5k. The plan starts with four to five days of running and includes VO_2 max and tempo runs in the first week. If you have not been running for at least six months, start with the Noncompetitive Novices plan.

Running Your First 10k (see page 132): This 12-week plan is designed for runners who have been training for six to nine months and are comfortable running 20 miles per week. If you haven't been training for at least six months, or aren't comfortable at 20 miles per week, you should start with the Noncompetitive Intermediate Runners plan.

Running Your First Half Marathon (see page 138): To begin this 12-week plan, you should be comfortable running 20 to 25 miles per week and be able to complete at least an 8-mile run.

Running Your First Marathon (see page 144): This 12-week plan is designed for seasoned runners who have been running for more than a year, are comfortable running over 25 miles per week, and are ready to begin with long runs starting at 14 miles, leading up to a full marathon.

New Runners Training Plan

		WORKOUT	RUN DETAIL	STRENGTH	STRETCHING
WEEK 1	**M**	Rest or Cross-Training	Rest or 30 minutes cross-training	CR (pg. 79)	
	Tu	Easy	Run 3 minutes; walk 5 minutes. Repeat 3 times for a total of 24 minutes.	LB (pg. 79)	PR (pg. 21)
	W	Rest Day	Rest		
	Th	Easy	Run 2 minutes; walk 4 minutes. Repeat 4 times for a total of 24 minutes.	HP (pg. 80)	SR (pg. 33)
	F	Rest Day	Rest	GS (pg. 80)	SS (pg. 43) or AS (pg. 49)
	Sa	Rest or Cross-Training	Rest or 30 minutes cross-training		
	Su	Easy	Run 4 minutes; walk 5 minutes. Repeat 3 times for a total of 27 minutes.	PD (pg. 66)	SS (pg. 43) or AS (pg. 49)
WEEK 2	**M**	Rest or Cross-Training	Rest or 30 minutes cross-training	CR (pg. 79)	
	Tu	Easy	Run 3 minutes; walk 7 minutes. Repeat 3 times for a total of 30 minutes.	LB (pg. 79)	SS (pg. 43) or AS (pg. 49)
	W	Rest or Cross-Training	Rest or 30 minutes cross-training		
	Th	Easy	Run 2 minutes; walk 8 minutes. Repeat 3 times for a total of 30 minutes.	HP (pg. 80)	PR (pg. 21)
	F	Rest Day	Rest	GS (pg. 80)	SR (pg. 33)
	Sa	Rest or Cross-Training	Rest or 30 minutes cross-training		
	Su	Easy	Run 3 minutes; walk 9 minutes. Repeat 3 times for a total of 36 minutes.	PD (pg. 66)	SS (pg. 43) or AS (pg. 49)

Continued

		WORKOUT	RUN DETAIL	STRENGTH	STRETCHING
WEEK 3	**M**	Rest Day	Rest	CR (pg. 79)	
	Tu	Easy	Run 3 minutes; walk 8 minutes. Repeat 3 times for a total of 33 minutes.	LB (pg. 79)	SS (pg. 43) or AS (pg. 49)
	W	Rest or Cross-Training	Rest or 30 minutes cross-training		
	Th	Easy	Run 2 minutes; walk 7 minutes. Repeat 4 times for a total of 36 minutes.	HP (pg. 80)	PR (pg. 21)
	F	Rest Day	Rest	GS (pg. 80)	SR (pg. 33)
	Sa	Rest or Cross-Training	Rest or 30 minutes cross-training		
	Su	Easy	Run 4 minutes; walk 6 minutes. Repeat 4 times for a total of 40 minutes.	QR (pg. 66)	SS (pg. 43) or AS (pg. 49)
WEEK 4	**M**	Rest Day	Rest	CR (pg. 79)	SR (pg. 33)
	Tu	Easy	Run 4 minutes; walk 6 minutes. Repeat 4 times for a total of 40 minutes.	LB (pg. 79)	SS (pg. 43) or AS (pg. 49)
	W	Rest or Cross-Training	Rest or 30 minutes cross-training		
	Th	Easy	Run 4 minutes; walk 7 minutes. Repeat 4 times for a total of 44 minutes.	HP (pg. 80)	PR (pg. 21)
	F	Rest Day	Rest	GS (pg. 80)	SR (pg. 33)
	Sa	Rest or Cross-Training	Rest or 30 minutes cross-training		
	Su	Easy	Run 2 minutes; walk 7 minutes. Repeat 5 times for a total of 45 minutes.	PD (pg. 66)	SS (pg. 43) or AS (pg. 49)

		WORKOUT	RUN DETAIL	STRENGTH	STRETCHING
WEEK 5	**M**	Rest Day	Rest	CR (pg. 79)	PR (pg. 21)
	Tu	Easy	Run 4 minutes; walk 6 minutes. Repeat 4 times for a total of 40 minutes.	LB (pg. 79)	SS (pg. 43) or AS (pg. 49)
	W	Rest or Cross-Training	Rest or 30 minutes cross-training		
	Th	Easy	Run 5 minutes; walk 9 minutes. Repeat 3 times for a total of 42 minutes.	HP (pg. 80)	PR (pg. 21)
	F	Rest Day	Rest	GS (pg. 80)	SR (pg. 33)
	Sa	Rest or Cross-Training	Rest or 30 minutes cross-training		
	Su	Easy	Run 3 minutes; walk 8 minutes. Repeat 4 times for a total of 44 minutes.	PD (pg. 66)	SS (pg. 43) or AS (pg. 49)
WEEK 6	**M**	Rest Day	Rest	CR (pg. 79)	SR (pg. 33)
	Tu	Easy	Run 4 minutes; walk 5 minutes. Repeat 5 times for a total of 45 minutes.	LB (pg. 79)	SS (pg. 43) or AS (pg. 49)
	W	Rest or Cross-Training	Rest or 30 minutes cross-training		
	Th	Easy	Run 6 minutes; walk 4 minutes. Repeat 4 times for a total of 40 minutes.	HP (pg. 80)	PR (pg. 21)
	F	Rest Day	Rest	GS (pg. 80)	SR (pg. 33)
	Sa	Rest or Cross-Training	Rest or 30 minutes cross-training		
	Su	Easy	Run 3 minutes; walk 7 minutes. Repeat 5 times for a total of 50 minutes.	QR (pg. 66)	SS (pg. 43) or AS (pg. 49)

NEW RUNNERS TRAINING PLAN

Continued

		WORKOUT	RUN DETAIL	STRENGTH	STRETCHING
WEEK 7	**M**	Rest Day	Rest	CR (pg. 79)	PR (pg. 21)
	Tu	Easy	Run 5 minutes; walk 5 minutes. Repeat 4 times for a total of 40 minutes.	LB (pg. 79)	SS (pg. 43) or AS (pg. 49)
	W	Rest or Cross-Training	Rest or 30 minutes cross-training		
	Th	Easy	Run 6 minutes; walk 3 minutes. Repeat 5 times for a total of 45 minutes.	HP (pg. 80)	PR (pg. 21)
	F	Rest Day	Rest	PL (pg. 80)	SR (pg. 33)
	Sa	Rest or Cross-Training	Rest or 30 minutes cross-training		
	Su	Easy	Run 4 minutes; walk 9 minutes. Repeat 3 times for a total of 39 minutes.	PD (pg. 66)	SS (pg. 43) or AS (pg. 49)
WEEK 8	**M**	Rest Day	Rest	CR (pg. 79)	SR (pg. 33)
	Tu	Easy	Run 6 minutes; walk 5 minutes. Repeat 4 times for a total of 44 minutes.	LB (pg. 79)	SS (pg. 43) or AS (pg. 49)
	W	Rest or Cross-Training	Rest or 30 minutes cross-training		
	Th	Easy	Run 6 minutes; walk 3 minutes. Repeat 4 times for a total of 36 minutes.	HP (pg. 80)	PR (pg. 21)
	F	Rest Day	Rest	PL (pg. 80)	SR (pg. 33)
	Sa	Rest or Cross-Training	Rest or 30 minutes cross-training		
	Su	Easy	Run 4 minutes; walk 8 minutes. Repeat 5 times for a total of 60 minutes.	QR (pg. 66)	SS (pg. 43) or AS (pg. 49)

NEW RUNNERS TRAINING PLAN

		WORKOUT	RUN DETAIL	STRENGTH	STRETCHING
WEEK 9	M	Rest Day	Rest	CR (pg. 79)	SR (pg. 33)
	Tu	Easy	Run 8 minutes; walk 1 minute. Repeat 3 times for a total of 27 minutes.	LB (pg. 79)	SS (pg. 43) or AS (pg. 49)
	W	Rest or Cross-Training	Rest or 30 minutes cross-training		
	Th	Easy	Run 7 minutes; walk 4 minutes. Repeat 4 times for a total of 44 minutes.	HP (pg. 80)	PR (pg. 21)
	F	Rest Day	Rest	PL (pg. 80)	SR (pg. 33)
	Sa	Rest or Cross-Training	Rest or 30 minutes cross-training		
	Su	Easy	Run 5 minutes; walk 7 minutes. Repeat 3 times for a total of 36 minutes.	QR (pg. 66)	SS (pg. 43) or AS (pg. 49)
WEEK 10	M	Rest Day	Rest	CR (pg. 79)	SR (pg. 33)
	Tu	Easy	2 miles easy, walk 3 minutes, 1 mile easy	LB (pg. 79)	SS (pg. 43) or AS (pg. 49)
	W	Rest or Cross-Training	Rest or 30 minutes cross-training		
	Th	Easy	3 miles easy	HP (pg. 80)	PR (pg. 21)
	F	Rest Day	Rest	PL (pg. 80)	SR (pg. 33)
	Sa	Rest or Cross-Training	Rest or 30 minutes cross-training		
	Su	Easy	Run 8 minutes; walk 2 minutes. Repeat 5 times for a total of 50 minutes.	PD (pg. 66)	SS (pg. 43) or AS (pg. 49)

NEW RUNNERS TRAINING PLAN

Noncompetitive Novices Training Plan

		WORKOUT	RUN DETAIL	STRENGTH	STRETCHING
WEEK 1	**M**	Rest or Cross-Training	Rest or 30 minutes cross-training	CR (pg. 79)	
	Tu	Easy	3 miles easy	LB (pg. 79)	PR (pg. 21)
	W	Rest or Cross-Training	Rest or 30 minutes cross-training		
	Th	Easy	2 miles easy	HP (pg. 80)	SR (pg. 33)
	F	Easy	3 miles easy	GS (pg. 80)	SS (pg. 43) or AS (pg. 49)
	Sa	Rest or Cross-Training	Rest or 30 minutes cross-training		
	Su	Long	4-mile run	PD (pg. 66)	SS (pg. 43) or AS (pg. 49)
WEEK 2	**M**	Rest or Cross-Training	Rest or 30 minutes cross-training	CR (pg. 79)	
	Tu	Threshold Interval	4 x 800 meters with 60 seconds rest	LB (pg. 79)	SS (pg. 43) or AS (pg. 49)
	W	Rest or Cross-Training	Rest or 30 minutes cross-training		
	Th	Easy	2 miles easy	HP (pg. 80)	PR (pg. 21)
	F	Short Tempo	3 miles tempo	GS (pg. 80)	SR (pg. 33)
	Sa	Rest or Cross-Training	Rest or 30 minutes cross-training		
	Su	Long	5-mile run	PD (pg. 66)	SS (pg. 43) or AS (pg. 49)

NONCOMPETITIVE NOVICES TRAINING PLAN

		WORKOUT	RUN DETAIL	STRENGTH	STRETCHING
WEEK 3	**M**	Rest or Cross-Training	Rest or 30 minutes cross-training	CR (pg. 79)	
	Tu	VO₂ Max	8 x 400 meters with 2 minutes rest	LB (pg. 79)	SS (pg. 43) or AS (pg. 49)
	W	Rest or Cross-Training	Rest or 30 minutes cross-training		
	Th	Easy	3 miles easy	HP (pg. 80)	PR (pg. 21)
	F	Short Tempo	3 miles tempo	GS (pg. 80)	SR (pg. 33)
	Sa	Rest or Cross-Training	Rest or 30 minutes cross-training		
	Su	Long	5-mile run	QR (pg. 66)	SS (pg. 43) or AS (pg. 49)
WEEK 4	**M**	Rest or Cross-Training	Rest or 30 minutes cross-training	CR (pg. 79)	SR (pg. 33)
	Tu	Hill Repeats	5 x 60 seconds uphill with 2 minutes rest	LB (pg. 79)	SS (pg. 43) or AS (pg. 49)
	W	Rest or Cross-Training	Rest or 30 minutes cross-training		
	Th	Easy	3 miles easy	HP (pg. 80)	PR (pg. 21)
	F	Tempo Interval	2 x 2 miles with 3 minutes rest	GS (pg. 80)	SR (pg. 33)
	Sa	Rest or Cross-Training	Rest or 30 minutes cross-training		
	Su	Long	6-mile run	PD (pg. 66)	SS (pg. 43) or AS (pg. 49)

Continued

		WORKOUT	RUN DETAIL	STRENGTH	STRETCHING
WEEK 5	M	Rest or Cross-Training	Rest or 30 minutes cross-training	CR (pg. 79)	PR (pg. 21)
	Tu	Threshold Interval	6 x 800 meters with 60 seconds rest	LB (pg. 79)	SS (pg. 43) or AS (pg. 49)
	W	Rest or Cross-Training	Rest or 30 minutes cross-training		
	Th	Easy	3 miles easy	HP (pg. 80)	PR (pg. 21)
	F	Long Tempo	4 miles tempo	GS (pg. 80)	SR (pg. 33)
	Sa	Rest or Cross-Training	Rest or 30 minutes cross-training		
	Su	Long	6-mile run	QR (pg. 66)	SS (pg. 43) or AS (pg. 49)
WEEK 6	M	Rest or Cross-Training	Rest or 30 minutes cross-training	CR (pg. 79)	SR (pg. 33)
	Tu	VO$_2$ max	10 x 400 meters with 2 minutes rest	LB (pg. 79)	SS (pg. 43) or AS (pg. 49)
	W	Rest or Cross-Training	Rest or 30 minutes cross-training		
	Th	Easy	4 miles easy	HP (pg. 80)	PR (pg. 21)
	F	Tempo Interval	2 x 2.5 miles with 3 minutes rest	GS (pg. 80)	SR (pg. 33)
	Sa	Rest or Cross-Training	Rest or 30 minutes cross-training		
	Su	Long	6-mile run	PD (pg. 66)	SS (pg. 43) or AS (pg. 49)

		WORKOUT	RUN DETAIL	STRENGTH	STRETCHING
WEEK 7	M	Rest or Cross-Training	Rest or 30 minutes cross-training	CR (pg. 79)	PR (pg. 21)
	Tu	Hill Repeats	6 x 60 seconds uphill with 2 minutes rest	LB (pg. 79)	SS (pg. 43) or AS (pg. 49)
	W	Rest or Cross-Training	Rest or 30 minutes cross-training		
	Th	Easy	4 miles easy	HP (pg. 80)	PR (pg. 21)
	F	Long Tempo	5 miles tempo	PL (pg. 80)	SR (pg. 33)
	Sa	Rest or Cross-Training	Rest or 30 minutes cross-training		
	Su	Long	6-mile run	QR (pg. 66)	SS (pg. 43) or AS (pg. 49)
WEEK 8	M	Rest or Cross-Training	Rest or 30 minutes cross-training	CR (pg. 79)	SR (pg. 33)
	Tu	Threshold Interval	6 x 1,000 meters with 60 seconds rest	LB (pg. 79)	SS (pg. 43) or AS (pg. 49)
	W	Rest or Cross-Training	Rest or 30 minutes cross-training		
	Th	Easy	4 miles easy	HP (pg. 80)	PR (pg. 21)
	F	Short Tempo	3 miles tempo	PL (pg. 80)	SR (pg. 33)
	Sa	Rest or Cross-Training	Rest or 30 minutes cross-training		
	Su	Long	7-mile run	PD (pg. 66)	SS (pg. 43) or AS (pg. 49)

Noncompetitive Intermediate Runners Training Plan

		WORKOUT	RUN DETAIL	STRENGTH	STRETCHING
WEEK 1	M	Rest or Cross-Training	Rest or 30 minutes cross-training	CR (pg. 79)	
	Tu	Short Tempo	2 miles tempo	LB (pg. 79)	PR (pg. 21)
	W	Rest or Cross-Training	Rest or 30 minutes cross-training		
	Th	Easy	4 miles easy	HP (pg. 80)	SR (pg. 33)
	F	Easy	3 miles easy	GS (pg. 80)	SS (pg. 43) or AS (pg. 49)
	Sa	Rest or Cross-Training	Rest or 30 minutes cross-training		
	Su	Long	6-mile run	PD (pg. 66)	SS (pg. 43) or AS (pg. 49)
WEEK 2	M	Rest or Cross-Training	Rest or 30 minutes cross-training	CR (pg. 79)	
	Tu	VO$_2$ Max	8 x 400 meters with 2 minutes rest	LB (pg. 79)	SS (pg. 43) or AS (pg. 49)
	W	Rest or Cross-Training	Rest or 30 minutes cross-training		
	Th	Easy	3 miles easy	HP (pg. 80)	PR (pg. 21)
	F	Tempo Interval	2 x 2 miles with 3 minutes rest	GS (pg. 80)	SR (pg. 33)
	Sa	Rest or Cross-Training	Rest or 30 minutes cross-training		
	Su	Long	6-mile run	QR (pg. 66)	SS (pg. 43) or AS (pg. 49)

		WORKOUT	RUN DETAIL	STRENGTH	STRETCHING
WEEK 3	**M**	Rest or Cross-Training	Rest or 30 minutes cross-training	CR (pg. 79)	
	Tu	Hill Repeats	6 x 60 seconds uphill with 2 minutes rest	LB (pg. 79)	SS (pg. 43) or AS (pg. 49)
	W	Rest or Cross-Training	Rest or 30 minutes cross-training		
	Th	Easy	3 miles easy	HP (pg. 80)	PR (pg. 21)
	F	Long Tempo	5 miles tempo	GS (pg. 80)	SR (pg. 33)
	Sa	Rest or Cross-Training	Rest or 30 minutes cross-training		
	Su	Long	7-mile run	QR (pg. 66)	SS (pg. 43) or AS (pg. 49)
WEEK 4	**M**	Rest or Cross-Training	Rest or 30 minutes cross-training	CR (pg. 79)	SR (pg. 33)
	Tu	VO₂ Max	6 x 800 meters with 4 minutes rest	LB (pg. 79)	SS (pg. 43) or AS (pg. 49)
	W	Rest or Cross-Training	Rest or 30 minutes cross-training		
	Th	Easy	3 miles easy	HP (pg. 80)	PR (pg. 21)
	F	Tempo Interval	2 x 2.5 miles with 3 minutes rest	GS (pg. 80)	SR (pg. 33)
	Sa	Rest or Cross-Training	Rest or 30 minutes cross-training		
	Su	Long	7-mile run	PD (pg. 66)	SS (pg. 43) or AS (pg. 49)

NONCOMPETITIVE INTERMEDIATE RUNNERS TRAINING PLAN

Continued

		WORKOUT	RUN DETAIL	STRENGTH	STRETCHING
WEEK 5	M	Rest or Cross-Training	Rest or 30 minutes cross-training	CR (pg. 79)	PR (pg. 21)
	Tu	Threshold Interval	4 x 1 mile with 90 seconds rest	LB (pg. 79)	SS (pg. 43) or AS (pg. 49)
	W	Rest or Cross-Training	Rest or 30 minutes cross-training		
	Th	Easy	3 miles easy	HP (pg. 80)	PR (pg. 21)
	F	Long Tempo	5 miles tempo	GS (pg. 80)	SR (pg. 33)
	Sa	Rest or Cross-Training	Rest or 30 minutes cross-training		
	Su	Long	7-mile run	QR (pg. 66)	SS (pg. 43) or AS (pg. 49)
WEEK 6	M	Rest or Cross-Training	Rest or 30 minutes cross-training	CR (pg. 79)	SR (pg. 33)
	Tu	Hill Repeats	8 x 60 seconds uphill with 2 minutes rest	LB (pg. 79)	SS (pg. 43) or AS (pg. 49)
	W	Rest or Cross-Training	Rest or 30 minutes cross-training		
	Th	Easy	4 miles easy	HP (pg. 80)	PR (pg. 21)
	F	Short Tempo	3 miles tempo	GS (pg. 80)	SR (pg. 33)
	Sa	Rest or Cross-Training	Rest or 30 minutes cross-training		
	Su	Long	8-mile run	PD (pg. 66)	SS (pg. 43) or AS (pg. 49)

		WORKOUT	RUN DETAIL	STRENGTH	STRETCHING
WEEK 7	**M**	Rest or Cross-Training	Rest or 30 minutes cross-training	CR (pg. 79)	PR (pg. 21)
	Tu	VO$_2$ Max	12 x 400 meters with 2 minutes rest	LB (pg. 79)	SS (pg. 43) or AS (pg. 49)
	W	Rest or Cross-Training	Rest or 30 minutes cross-training		
	Th	Easy	4 miles easy	HP (pg. 80)	PR (pg. 21)
	F	Tempo Interval	2 x 3 miles with 4 minutes rest	PL (pg. 80)	SR (pg. 33)
	Sa	Rest or Cross-Training	Rest or 30 minutes cross-training		
	Su	Long	8-mile run	QR (pg. 66)	SS (pg. 43) or AS (pg. 49)
WEEK 8	**M**	Rest or Cross-Training	Rest or 30 minutes cross-training	CR (pg. 79)	SR (pg. 33)
	Tu	Threshold Interval	8 x 1,000 meters with 60 seconds rest	LB (pg. 79)	SS (pg. 43) or AS (pg. 49)
	W	Rest or Cross-Training	Rest or 30 minutes cross-training		
	Th	Easy	4 miles easy	HP (pg. 80)	PR (pg. 21)
	F	Long Tempo	6 miles tempo	PL (pg. 80)	SR (pg. 33)
	Sa	Rest or Cross-Training	Rest or 30 minutes cross-training		
	Su	Long	9-mile run	PD (pg. 66)	SS (pg. 43) or AS (pg. 49)

NONCOMPETITIVE INTERMEDIATE RUNNERS TRAINING PLAN

Running Your First 5k Training Plan

		WORKOUT	RUN DETAIL	STRENGTH	STRETCHING
WEEK 1	**M**	Easy	3 miles easy	CR (pg. 79)	
	Tu	VO₂ Max	8 x 400 meters with 2 minutes rest	LB (pg. 79)	PR (pg. 21)
	W	Rest or Cross-Training	Rest or 30 minutes cross-training		
	Th	Easy or Cross-Training	3 miles easy or cross-training	HP (pg. 80)	SR (pg. 33)
	F	Short Tempo	3 miles tempo	GS (pg. 80)	SS (pg. 43) or AS (pg. 49)
	Sa	Rest or Cross Training	Rest or 30 minutes cross-training		
	Su	Long	4-mile run	QR (pg. 66)	SS (pg. 43) or AS (pg. 49)
WEEK 2	**M**	Easy	3 miles easy	CR (pg. 79)	
	Tu	Hill Repeats	6 x 60 seconds uphill with 2 minutes rest	LB (pg. 79)	PR (pg. 21)
	W	Rest or Cross-Training	Rest or 30 minutes cross-training		
	Th	Easy or Cross-Training	3 miles easy or cross-training	HP (pg. 80)	SR (pg. 33)
	F	Threshold Interval	5 x 1,000 meters with 90 seconds rest	GS (pg. 80)	SS (pg. 43) or AS (pg. 49)
	Sa	Rest or Cross-Training	Rest or 30 minutes cross-training		
	Su	Long	4-mile run	PD (pg. 66)	SS (pg. 43) or AS (pg. 49)

		WORKOUT	RUN DETAIL	STRENGTH	STRETCHING
WEEK 3	**M**	Easy	3 miles easy	CR (pg. 79)	
	Tu	Race Specific	8 x 400 meters with 45 seconds rest	LB (pg. 79)	PR (pg. 21)
	W	Rest or Cross-Training	Rest or 30 minutes cross-training		
	Th	Easy or Cross-Training	3 miles easy or cross-training	HP (pg. 80)	SR (pg. 33)
	F	Short Tempo	3 miles tempo	GS (pg. 80)	SS (pg. 43) or AS (pg. 49)
	Sa	Rest or Cross-Training	Rest or 30 minutes cross-training		
	Su	Long	5-mile run	QR (pg. 66)	SS (pg. 43) or AS (pg. 49)
WEEK 4	**M**	Easy	3 miles easy	CR (pg. 79)	
	Tu	Race Specific	4 x 800 meters with 45 seconds rest	LB (pg. 79)	PR (pg. 21)
	W	Rest or Cross-Training	Rest or 30 minutes cross-training		
	Th	Easy or Cross-Training	3 miles easy or cross-training	HP (pg. 80)	SR (pg. 33)
	F	Hill Repeats	8 x 60 seconds uphill with 2 minutes rest	GS (pg. 80)	SS (pg. 43) or AS (pg. 49)
	Sa	Rest or Cross-Training	Rest or 30 minutes cross-training		
	Su	Long	5-mile run	PD (pg. 66)	SS (pg. 43) or AS (pg. 49)

Continued

		WORKOUT	RUN DETAIL	STRENGTH	STRETCHING
WEEK 5	**M**	Easy	3 miles easy	CR (pg. 79)	PR (pg. 21)
	Tu	Race Specific	10 x 400 meters with 30 seconds rest	LB (pg. 79)	SS (pg. 43) or AS (pg. 49)
	W	Rest or Cross-Training	Rest or 30 minutes cross-training		
	Th	Easy or Cross-Training	3 miles easy or cross-training	HP (pg. 80)	PR (pg. 21)
	F	Tempo Interval	2 x 2 miles with 3 minutes rest	PL (pg. 80)	SR (pg. 33)
	Sa	Rest or Cross-Training	Rest or 30 minutes cross-training		
	Su	Long	6-mile run	QR (pg. 66)	SS (pg. 43) or AS (pg. 49)
WEEK 6	**M**	Easy	3 miles easy	CR (pg. 79)	PR (pg. 21)
	Tu	Race Specific	4 x 1,000 meters with 45 seconds rest	LB (pg. 79)	SS (pg. 43) or AS (pg. 49)
	W	Rest or Cross-Training	Rest or 30 minutes cross-training		
	Th	Easy or Cross-Training	3 miles easy or cross-training	HP (pg. 80)	PR (pg. 21)
	F	Long Tempo	4 miles tempo	PL (pg. 80)	SR (pg. 33)
	Sa	Rest or Cross-Training	Rest or 30 minutes cross-training		
	Su	Long	6-mile run	PD (pg. 66)	SS (pg. 43) or AS (pg. 49)

		WORKOUT	RUN DETAIL	STRENGTH	STRETCHING
WEEK 7	**M**	Easy	3 miles easy	CR (pg. 79)	PR (pg. 21)
	Tu	Race Specific	12 x 400 meters with 45 seconds rest	LB (pg. 79)	SS (pg. 43) or AS (pg. 49)
	W	Rest or Cross-Training	Rest or 30 minutes cross-training		
	Th	Easy or Cross-Training	3 miles easy or cross-training	HP (pg. 80)	PR (pg. 21)
	F	Short Tempo	3 miles tempo	PL (pg. 80)	SR (pg. 33)
	Sa	Rest or Cross-Training	Rest or 30 minutes cross-training		
	Su	Long	6-mile run	QR (pg. 66)	SS (pg. 43) or AS (pg. 49)
WEEK 8	**M**	Easy	3 miles easy	CR (pg. 79)	PR (pg. 21)
	Tu	Race Specific	6 x 800 meters with 60 seconds rest	LB (pg. 79)	SS (pg. 43) or AS (pg. 49)
	W	Rest or Cross-Training	Rest or 30 minutes cross-training		
	Th	Rest or Cross-Training	Rest or 30 minutes cross-training	HP (pg. 80)	PR (pg. 21)
	F	Tempo Interval	2 x 2.5 miles with 3 minutes rest	PL (pg. 80)	SR (pg. 33)
	Sa	Rest or Cross-Training	Rest or 30 minutes cross-training		
	Su	Long	7-mile run	PD (pg. 66)	SS (pg. 43) or AS (pg. 49)

Continued

		WORKOUT	RUN DETAIL	STRENGTH	STRETCHING
WEEK 9	M	Easy	3 miles easy	CR (pg. 79)	PR (pg. 21)
	Tu	Race Specific	12 x 400 meters with 30 seconds rest	LB (pg. 79)	SS (pg. 43) or AS (pg. 49)
	W	Rest or Cross-Training	Rest or 30 minutes cross-training		
	Th	Easy or Cross-Training	3 miles easy or cross-training	HP (pg. 80)	PR (pg. 21)
	F	Hill Repeats	7 x 60 seconds uphill with 2 minutes rest	PL (pg. 80)	SR (pg. 33)
	Sa	Rest or Cross-Training	Rest or 30 minutes cross-training		
	Su	Long	7-mile run	QR (pg. 66)	SS (pg. 43) or AS (pg. 49)
WEEK 10	M	Easy	3 miles easy	CR (pg. 79)	PR (pg. 21)
	Tu	Race Specific	6 x 800 meters with 45 seconds rest	LB (pg. 79)	SS (pg. 43) or AS (pg. 49)
	W	Rest or Cross-Training	Rest or 30 minutes cross-training		
	Th	Easy or Cross-Training	3 miles easy or cross-training	HP (pg. 80)	PR (pg. 21)
	F	Long Tempo	4 miles tempo	PL (pg. 80)	SR (pg. 33)
	Sa	Rest or Cross-Training	Rest or 30 minutes cross-training		
	Su	Long	7-mile run	PD (pg. 66)	SS (pg. 43) or AS (pg. 49)

		WORKOUT	RUN DETAIL	STRENGTH	STRETCHING
WEEK 11	**M**	Easy	3 miles easy	CR (pg. 79)	PR (pg. 21)
	Tu	Race Specific	5 x 1,000 meters with 45 seconds rest	LB (pg. 79)	SS (pg. 43) or AS (pg. 49)
	W	Rest or Cross-Training	Rest or 30 minutes cross-training		
	Th	Easy	3 miles easy	HP (pg. 80)	PR (pg. 21)
	F	Short Tempo	2 miles tempo	PL (pg. 80)	SR (pg. 33)
	Sa	Rest or Cross-Training	Rest or 30 minutes cross-training		
	Su	Easy	3 miles easy	QR (pg. 66)	SS (pg. 43) or AS (pg. 49)
WEEK 12	**M**	Easy	3 miles easy	CR (pg. 79)	PR (pg. 21)
	Tu	VO$_2$ Max	8 x 400 meters with 2 minutes rest	LB (pg. 79)	SS (pg. 43) or AS (pg. 49)
	W	Rest or Cross-Training	Rest or 30 minutes cross-training		
	Th	Easy	3 miles easy	QR (pg. 66)	PR (pg. 21)
	F	Rest Day	Rest		
	Sa	Easy	2 miles easy		AS (pg. 49)
	Su	Race Day	Race Day		

Running Your First 10k Training Plan

		WORKOUT	RUN DETAIL	STRENGTH	STRETCHING
WEEK 1	**M**	Easy	3 miles easy	CR (pg. 79)	
	Tu	VO₂ Max	10 x 400 meters with 2 minutes rest	LB (pg. 79)	PR (pg. 21)
	W	Rest or Cross-Training	Rest or 30 minutes cross-training		
	Th	Easy	3 miles easy	HP (pg. 80)	SR (pg. 33)
	F	Short Tempo	3 miles tempo	GS (pg. 80)	SS (pg. 43) or AS (pg. 49)
	Sa	Rest or Cross-Training	Rest or 30 minutes cross-training		
	Su	Long	5-mile run	PD (pg. 66)	SS (pg. 43) or AS (pg. 49)
WEEK 2	**M**	Easy	3 miles easy	CR (pg. 79)	
	Tu	Hill Repeats	8 x 60 seconds uphill with 2 minutes rest	LB (pg. 79)	PR (pg. 21)
	W	Rest or Cross-Training	Rest or 30 minutes cross-training		
	Th	Easy	3 miles easy	HP (pg. 80)	SR (pg. 33)
	F	Threshold Interval	5 x 1,000 meters with 90 seconds rest	GS (pg. 80)	SS (pg. 43) or AS (pg. 49)
	Sa	Rest or Cross-Training	Rest or 30 minutes cross-training		
	Su	Long	6-mile run	QR (pg. 66)	SS (pg. 43) or AS (pg. 49)

		WORKOUT	RUN DETAIL	STRENGTH	STRETCHING
WEEK 3	**M**	Easy	3 miles easy	CR (pg. 79)	
	Tu	Race Specific	16 x 400 meters with 45 seconds rest	LB (pg. 79)	PR (pg. 21)
	W	Rest or Cross-Training	Rest or 30 minutes cross-training		
	Th	Easy	3 miles easy	HP (pg. 80)	SR (pg. 33)
	F	Long Tempo	4 miles tempo	GS (pg. 80)	SS (pg. 43) or AS (pg. 49)
	Sa	Rest or Cross-Training	Rest or 30 minutes cross-training		
	Su	Long	6-mile run	PD (pg. 66)	SS (pg. 43) or AS (pg. 49)
WEEK 4	**M**	Easy	3 miles easy	CR (pg. 79)	
	Tu	Race Specific	10 x 800 meters with 60 seconds rest	LB (pg. 79)	PR (pg. 21)
	W	Rest or Cross-Training	Rest or 30 minutes cross-training		
	Th	Easy	3 miles easy	HP (pg. 80)	SR (pg. 33)
	F	Tempo Interval	2 x 2 miles with 3 minutes rest	GS (pg. 80)	SS (pg. 43) or AS (pg. 49)
	Sa	Rest or Cross-Training	Rest or 30 minutes cross-training		
	Su	Long	7-mile run	QR (pg. 66)	SS (pg. 43) or AS (pg. 49)

Continued

		WORKOUT	RUN DETAIL	STRENGTH	STRETCHING
WEEK 5	**M**	Easy	3 miles easy	CR (pg. 79)	PR (pg. 21)
	Tu	Race Specific	8 x 1,000 meters with 60 seconds rest	LB (pg. 79)	SS (pg. 43) or AS (pg. 49)
	W	Rest or Cross-Training	Rest or 30 minutes cross-training		
	Th	Easy	5 miles easy	HP (pg. 80)	PR (pg. 21)
	F	Hill Repeats	8 x 60 seconds uphill with 2 minutes rest	PL (pg. 80)	SR (pg. 33)
	Sa	Rest or Cross-Training	Rest or 30 minutes cross-training		
	Su	Long	7-mile run	PD (pg. 66)	SS (pg. 43) or AS (pg. 49)
WEEK 6	**M**	Easy	3 miles easy	CR (pg. 79)	PR (pg. 21)
	Tu	Race Specific	4 x 1 mile with 60 seconds rest	LB (pg. 79)	SS (pg. 43) or AS (pg. 49)
	W	Rest or Cross-Training	Rest or 30 minutes cross-training		
	Th	Easy	3 miles easy	HP (pg. 80)	PR (pg. 21)
	F	Long Tempo	4 miles tempo	PL (pg. 80)	SR (pg. 33)
	Sa	Rest or Cross-Training	Rest or 30 minutes cross-training		
	Su	Long	7-mile run	QR (pg. 66)	SS (pg. 43) or AS (pg. 49)

		WORKOUT	RUN DETAIL	STRENGTH	STRETCHING
WEEK 7	**M**	Easy	3 miles easy	CR (pg. 79)	PR (pg. 21)
	Tu	Race Specific	16 x 400 meters with 30 seconds rest	LB (pg. 79)	SS (pg. 43) or AS (pg. 49)
	W	Rest or Cross-Training	Rest or 30 minutes cross-training		
	Th	Easy	3 miles easy	HP (pg. 80)	PR (pg. 21)
	F	VO$_2$ Max	3 x 1 mile with 4 minutes rest	PL (pg. 80)	SR (pg. 33)
	Sa	Rest or Cross-Training	Rest or 30 minutes cross-training		
	Su	Long	8-mile run	PD (pg. 66)	SS (pg. 43) or AS (pg. 49)
WEEK 8	**M**	Easy	3 miles easy	CR (pg. 79)	PR (pg. 21)
	Tu	Race Specific	10 x 800 meters with 45 seconds rest	LB (pg. 79)	SS (pg. 43) or AS (pg. 49)
	W	Rest or Cross-Training	Rest or 30 minutes cross-training		
	Th	Easy	3 miles easy	HP (pg. 80)	PR (pg. 21)
	F	Tempo Interval	2 x 2.5 miles with 3 minutes rest	PL (pg. 80)	SR (pg. 33)
	Sa	Rest or Cross-Training	Rest or 30 minutes cross-training		
	Su	Long	8-mile run	QR (pg. 66)	SS (pg. 43) or AS (pg. 49)

Continued

		WORKOUT	RUN DETAIL	STRENGTH	STRETCHING
WEEK 9	M	Easy	3 miles easy	CR (pg. 79)	PR (pg. 21)
	Tu	Race Specific	8 x 1,000 meters with 45 seconds rest	LB (pg. 79)	SS (pg. 43) or AS (pg. 49)
	W	Rest or Cross-Training	Rest or 30 minutes cross-training		
	Th	Easy	3 miles easy	HP (pg. 80)	PR (pg. 21)
	F	Long Tempo	5 miles tempo	PL (pg. 80)	SR (pg. 33)
	Sa	Rest or Cross-Training	Rest or 30 minutes cross-training		
	Su	Long	8-mile run	PD (pg. 66)	SS (pg. 43) or AS (pg. 49)
WEEK 10	M	Easy	3 miles easy	CR (pg. 79)	PR (pg. 21)
	Tu	Race Specific	4 x 1 mile with 60 seconds rest	LB (pg. 79)	SS (pg. 43) or AS (pg. 49)
	W	Rest or Cross-Training	Rest or 30 minutes cross-training		
	Th	Easy	3 miles easy	HP (pg. 80)	PR (pg. 21)
	F	VO$_2$ Max	10 x 400 meters with 2 minutes rest	PL (pg. 80)	SR (pg. 33)
	Sa	Rest or Cross-Training	30 minutes cross-training		
	Su	Long	9-mile run	QR (pg. 66)	SS (pg. 43) or AS (pg. 49)

		WORKOUT	RUN DETAIL	STRENGTH	STRETCHING
WEEK 11	**M**	Easy	3 miles easy	CR (pg. 79)	PR (pg. 21)
	Tu	Race Specific	2 x 2 miles with 60 seconds rest	LB (pg. 79)	SS (pg. 43) or AS (pg. 49)
	W	Rest or Cross-Training	Rest or 30 minutes cross-training		
	Th	Easy	3 miles easy	HP (pg. 80)	PR (pg. 21)
	F	Short Tempo	3 miles tempo	PL (pg. 80)	SR (pg. 33)
	Sa	Rest or Cross-Training	Rest or 30 minutes cross-training		
	Su	Easy	4 miles easy	PD (pg. 66)	SS (pg. 43) or AS (pg. 49)
WEEK 12	**M**	Easy	3 miles easy	CR (pg. 79)	PR (pg. 21)
	Tu	VO$_2$ Max	8 x 400 meters with 2 minutes rest	LB (pg. 79)	SS (pg. 43) or AS (pg. 49)
	W	Rest or Cross-Training	Rest or 30 minutes cross-training		
	Th	Easy	3 miles easy	QR (pg. 66)	PR (pg. 21)
	F	Rest Day	Rest		
	Sa	Easy	2 miles easy		AS (pg. 49)
	Su	Race Day	Race Day		

Running Your First Half Marathon Training Plan

		WORKOUT	RUN DETAIL	STRENGTH	STRETCHING
WEEK 1	M	Easy	3 miles easy	CR (pg. 79)	
	Tu	Hill Repeats	8 x 60 seconds uphill with 2 minutes rest	LB (pg. 79)	PR (pg. 21)
	W	Rest or Cross-Training	Rest or 30 minutes cross-training		
	Th	Easy	3 miles easy	HP (pg. 80)	SR (pg. 33)
	F	Short Tempo	3 miles tempo	GS (pg. 80)	SS (pg. 43) or AS (pg. 49)
	Sa	Rest or Cross-Training	Rest or 30 minutes cross-training		
	Su	Long	8-mile run	PD (pg. 66)	SS (pg. 43) or AS (pg. 49)
WEEK 2	M	Easy	3 miles easy	CR (pg. 79)	
	Tu	VO$_2$ Max	3 x 1 mile with 4 minutes rest	LB (pg. 79)	PR (pg. 21)
	W	Rest or Cross-Training	Rest or 30 minutes cross-training		
	Th	Easy	3 miles easy	HP (pg. 80)	SR (pg. 33)
	F	Short Tempo	4 miles tempo	GS (pg. 80)	SS (pg. 43) or AS (pg. 49)
	Sa	Rest or Cross-Training	Rest or 30 minutes cross-training		
	Su	Long	8-mile run	QR (pg. 66)	SS (pg. 43) or AS (pg. 49)

		WORKOUT	RUN DETAIL	STRENGTH	STRETCHING
WEEK 3	**M**	Easy	3 miles easy	CR (pg. 79)	
	Tu	Race Specific	5 x 1 mile with 60 seconds rest	LB (pg. 79)	PR (pg. 21)
	W	Rest or Cross-Training	Rest or 30 minutes cross-training		
	Th	Easy	3 miles easy	HP (pg. 80)	SR (pg. 33)
	F	Long Tempo	5 miles tempo	GS (pg. 80)	SS (pg. 43) or AS (pg. 49)
	Sa	Rest or Cross-Training	Rest or 30 minutes cross-training		
	Su	Long	9-mile run	PD (pg. 66)	SS (pg. 43) or AS (pg. 49)
WEEK 4	**M**	Easy	3 miles easy	CR (pg. 79)	
	Tu	Race Specific	5 x 1 mile with 60 seconds rest	LB (pg. 79)	PR (pg. 21)
	W	Rest or Cross-Training	Rest or 30 minutes cross-training		
	Th	Easy	3 miles easy	HP (pg. 80)	SR (pg. 33)
	F	Long Tempo	5 miles tempo	GS (pg. 80)	SS (pg. 43) or AS (pg. 49)
	Sa	Rest or Cross-Training	Rest or 30 minutes cross-training		
	Su	Long	9-mile run	PD (pg. 66)	SS (pg. 43) or AS (pg. 49)

Continued

		WORKOUT	RUN DETAIL	STRENGTH	STRETCHING
WEEK 5	**M**	Easy	3 miles easy	CR (pg. 79)	
	Tu	Race Specific	4 x 1.5 miles with 90 seconds rest	LB (pg. 79)	PR (pg. 21)
	W	Rest or Cross-Training	Rest or 30 minutes cross-training		
	Th	Easy	3 miles easy	HP (pg. 80)	SR (pg. 33)
	F	Short Tempo	4 miles tempo	GS (pg. 80)	SS (pg. 43) or AS (pg. 49)
	Sa	Rest or Cross-Training	Rest or 30 minutes cross-training		
	Su	Long	9-mile run	QR (pg. 66)	SS (pg. 43) or AS (pg. 49)
WEEK 6	**M**	Easy	3 miles easy	CR (pg. 79)	PR (pg. 21)
	Tu	Race Specific	3 x 2 miles with 2 minutes rest	LB (pg. 79)	SS (pg. 43) or AS (pg. 49)
	W	Rest or Cross-Training	Rest or 30 minutes cross-training		
	Th	Easy	5 miles easy	HP (pg. 80)	PR (pg. 21)
	F	Long Tempo	6 miles tempo	PL (pg. 80)	SR (pg. 33)
	Sa	Rest or Cross-Training	Rest or 30 minutes cross-training		
	Su	Long	10-mile run	PD (pg. 66)	SS (pg. 43) or AS (pg. 49)

		WORKOUT	RUN DETAIL	STRENGTH	STRETCHING
WEEK 7	**M**	Easy	3 miles easy	CR (pg. 79)	PR (pg. 21)
	Tu	Race Specific	6 x 1 mile with 90 seconds rest	LB (pg. 79)	SS (pg. 43) or AS (pg. 49)
	W	Rest or Cross-Training	Rest or 30 minutes cross-training		
	Th	Easy	3 miles easy	HP (pg. 80)	PR (pg. 21)
	F	Long Tempo	6 miles tempo	PL (pg. 80)	SR (pg. 33)
	Sa	Rest or Cross-Training	Rest or 30 minutes cross-training		
	Su	Long	12-mile run	PD (pg. 66)	SS (pg. 43) or AS (pg. 49)
WEEK 8	**M**	Easy	3 miles easy	CR (pg. 79)	PR (pg. 21)
	Tu	Race Specific	3 miles tempo, 2 minutes rest, 2 miles tempo, 2 minutes rest, 1 mile tempo	LB (pg. 79)	SS (pg. 43) or AS (pg. 49)
	W	Rest or Cross-Training	Rest or 30 minutes cross-training		
	Th	Easy	3 miles easy	HP (pg. 80)	PR (pg. 21)
	F	VO$_2$ Max	4 x 1 mile with 4 minutes rest	PL (pg. 80)	SR (pg. 33)
	Sa	Rest or Cross-Training	Rest or 30 minutes cross-training		
	Su	Long	12-mile run	QR (pg. 66)	SS (pg. 43) or AS (pg. 49)

Continued

		WORKOUT	RUN DETAIL	STRENGTH	STRETCHING
WEEK 9	**M**	Easy	3 miles easy	CR (pg. 79)	PR (pg. 21)
	Tu	Race Specific	4 x 1.5 miles with 90 seconds rest	LB (pg. 79)	SS (pg. 43) or AS (pg. 49)
	W	Rest or Cross-Training	Rest or 30 minutes cross-training		
	Th	Easy	3 miles easy	HP (pg. 80)	PR (pg. 21)
	F	Long Tempo	6 miles tempo	PL (pg. 80)	SR (pg. 33)
	Sa	Rest or Cross-Training	Rest or 30 minutes cross-training		
	Su	Long	14-mile run	PD (pg. 66)	SS (pg. 43) or AS (pg. 49)
WEEK 10	**M**	Easy	3 miles easy	CR (pg. 79)	PR (pg. 21)
	Tu	Race Specific	2 x 3 miles with 2 minutes rest	LB (pg. 79)	SS (pg. 43) or AS (pg. 49)
	W	Rest or Cross-Training	Rest or 30 minutes cross-training		
	Th	Easy	3 miles easy	HP (pg. 80)	PR (pg. 21)
	F	Hill Repeats	10 x 60 seconds uphill with 2 minutes rest	PL (pg. 80)	SR (pg. 33)
	Sa	Rest or Cross-Training	Rest or 30 minutes cross-training		
	Su	Long	14-mile run	QR (pg. 66)	SS (pg. 43) or AS (pg. 49)

		WORKOUT	RUN DETAIL	STRENGTH	STRETCHING
WEEK 11	**M**	Easy	3 miles easy	CR (pg. 79)	PR (pg. 21)
	Tu	Race Specific	3 x 2.5 miles with 2 minutes rest	LB (pg. 79)	SS (pg. 43) or AS (pg. 49)
	W	Rest or Cross-Training	Rest or 30 minutes cross-training		
	Th	Easy	3 miles easy	HP (pg. 80)	PR (pg. 21)
	F	Short Tempo	3 miles tempo	PL (pg. 80)	SR (pg. 33)
	Sa	Rest or Cross-Training	Rest or 30 minutes cross-training		
	Su	Easy	4 miles easy	PD (pg. 66)	SS (pg. 43) or AS (pg. 49)
WEEK 12	**M**	Easy	4 miles easy	CR (pg. 79)	PR (pg. 21)
	Tu	VO$_2$ Max	8 x 400 meters with 2 minutes rest	LB (pg. 79)	SS (pg. 43) or AS (pg. 49)
	W	Rest or Cross-Training	Rest or 30 minutes cross-training		
	Th	Easy	3 miles easy	QR (pg. 66)	PR (pg. 21)
	F	Rest Day	Rest		
	Sa	Easy	2 miles easy		AS (pg. 49)
	Su	Race Day	Race Day		

Running Your First Marathon Training Plan

		WORKOUT	RUN DETAIL	STRENGTH	STRETCHING
WEEK 1	**M**	Easy	3 miles easy	CR (pg. 79)	
	Tu	Tempo Interval	2 x 2 miles with 3 minutes rest	LB (pg. 79)	PR (pg. 21)
	W	Rest or Cross-Training	Rest or 30 minutes cross-training		
	Th	Easy	3 miles easy	HP (pg. 80)	SR (pg. 33)
	F	Rest or Cross-Training	Rest or 30 minutes cross-training		
	Sa	Easy	5 miles easy	GS (pg. 80)	PR (pg. 21)
	Su	Long	14-mile run	PD (pg. 66)	SS (pg. 43) or AS (pg. 49)
WEEK 2	**M**	Easy	3 miles easy	CR (pg. 79)	
	Tu	Threshold Interval	4 x 1 mile with 90 seconds rest	LB (pg. 79)	PR (pg. 21)
	W	Rest or Cross-Training	Rest or 30 minutes cross-training		
	Th	Easy	3 miles easy	HP (pg. 80)	SR (pg. 33)
	F	Long Tempo	6 miles tempo	GS (pg. 80)	SS (pg. 43) or AS (pg. 49)
	Sa	Rest or Cross-Training	Rest or 30 minutes cross-training		
	Su	Long	9-mile run	QR (pg. 66)	SS (pg. 43) or AS (pg. 49)

		WORKOUT	RUN DETAIL	STRENGTH	STRETCHING
WEEK 3	**M**	Easy	3 miles easy	CR (pg. 79)	
	Tu	Short Tempo	3 miles tempo	LB (pg. 79)	PR (pg. 21)
	W	Rest or Cross-Training	Rest or 30 minutes cross-training		
	Th	Easy	3 miles easy	HP (pg. 80)	SR (pg. 33)
	F	Rest or Cross-Training	Rest or 30 minutes cross-training		
	Sa	Easy	5 miles easy	GS (pg. 80)	SR (pg. 33)
	Su	Long	16-mile run	QR (pg. 66)	SS (pg. 43) or AS (pg. 49)
WEEK 4	**M**	Easy	3 miles easy	CR (pg. 79)	PR (pg. 21)
	Tu	Tempo Interval	2 x 3 miles with 3 minutes rest	LB (pg. 79)	SS (pg. 43) or AS (pg. 49)
	W	Rest or Cross-Training	Rest or 30 minutes cross-training		
	Th	Easy	5 miles easy	HP (pg. 80)	PR (pg. 21)
	F	Long Tempo	7 miles tempo	PL (pg. 80)	SR (pg. 33)
	Sa	Rest or Cross-Training	Rest or 30 minutes cross-training		
	Su	Long	10-mile run	PD (pg. 66)	SS (pg. 43) or AS (pg. 49)

Continued

		WORKOUT	RUN DETAIL	STRENGTH	STRETCHING
WEEK 5	**M**	Easy	4 miles easy	CR (pg. 79)	
	Tu	Threshold Interval	5 x 1 mile with 90 seconds rest	LB (pg. 79)	PR (pg. 21)
	W	Rest or Cross-Training	Rest or 30 minutes cross-training		
	Th	Easy	4 miles easy	HP (pg. 80)	SR (pg. 33)
	F	Rest or Cross-Training	Rest or 30 minutes cross-training		
	Sa	Easy	4 miles easy	GS (pg. 80)	PR (pg. 21)
	Su	Long	18-mile run	QR (pg. 66)	SS (pg. 43) or AS (pg. 49)
WEEK 6	**M**	Rest Day	Rest	CR (pg. 79)	PR (pg. 21)
	Tu	Easy	5 miles easy	HP (pg. 80)	PR (pg. 21)
	W	Threshold Interval	5 x 1 mile with 90 seconds rest	LB (pg. 79)	SS (pg. 43) or AS (pg. 49)
	Th	Rest or Cross-Training	Rest or 30 minutes cross-training		
	F	Easy	5 miles easy	PL (pg. 80)	SR (pg. 33)
	Sa	Rest or Cross-Training	Rest or 30 minutes cross-training		
	Su	Long Tempo	7 miles tempo	PD (pg. 66)	SS (pg. 43) or AS (pg. 49)

		WORKOUT	RUN DETAIL	STRENGTH	STRETCHING
WEEK 7	**M**	Easy	3 miles easy	CR (pg. 79)	
	Tu	Hill Repeats	8 x 60 seconds uphill with 2 minutes rest	LB (pg. 79)	PR (pg. 21)
	W	Rest or Cross-Training	Rest or 30 minutes cross-training		
	Th	Easy	5 miles easy	HP (pg. 80)	SR (pg. 33)
	F	Rest or Cross-Training	Rest or 30 minutes cross-training		
	Sa	Easy	5 miles easy	GS (pg. 80)	SR (pg. 33)
	Su	Long	20-mile run	QR (pg. 66)	SS (pg. 43) or AS (pg. 49)
WEEK 8	**M**	Rest Day	Rest		
	Tu	Easy	5 miles easy	CR (pg. 79)	PR (pg. 21)
	W	Rest or Cross-Training	Rest or 30 minutes cross-training		
	Th	Long Tempo	8 miles tempo	LB (pg. 79)	SR (pg. 33)
	F	Rest or Cross-Training	Rest or 30 minutes cross-training		
	Sa	Easy	5 miles easy	HP (pg. 80)	PR (pg. 21)
	Su	Long	14-mile run	PD (pg. 66)	SS (pg. 43) or AS (pg. 49)

Continued

		WORKOUT	RUN DETAIL	STRENGTH	STRETCHING
WEEK 9	M	Easy	3 miles easy	CR (pg. 79)	
	Tu	Short Tempo	4 miles tempo	LB (pg. 79)	PR (pg. 21)
	W	Rest or Cross-Training	Rest or 30 minutes cross-training		
	Th	Easy	5 miles easy	GS (pg. 80)	SR (pg. 33)
	F	Rest or Cross-Training	Rest or 30 minutes cross-training		
	Sa	Easy	6 miles easy	HP (pg. 80)	SR (pg. 33)
	Su	Long	20-mile run	QR (pg. 66)	SS (pg. 43) or AS (pg. 49)
WEEK 10	M	Rest Day	Rest	CR (pg. 79)	PR (pg. 21)
	Tu	Easy	3 miles easy	LB (pg. 79)	SS (pg. 43) or AS (pg. 49)
	W	Rest or Cross-Training	Rest or 30 minutes cross-training		
	Th	Easy	3 miles easy	HP (pg. 80)	PR (pg. 21)
	F	Long Tempo	6 miles tempo	PL (pg. 80)	SR (pg. 33)
	Sa	Rest or Cross-Training	Rest or 30 minutes cross-training		
	Su	Long	14-mile run	PD (pg. 66)	SS (pg. 43) or AS (pg. 49)

		WORKOUT	RUN DETAIL	STRENGTH	STRETCHING
WEEK 11	**M**	Easy	3 miles easy	CR (pg. 79)	PR (pg. 21)
	Tu	Threshold Interval	4 x 1 mile with 90 seconds rest	LB (pg. 79)	SS (pg. 43) or AS (pg. 49)
	W	Rest or Cross-Training	Rest or 30 minutes cross-training		
	Th	Easy	3 miles easy	HP (pg. 80)	PR (pg. 21)
	F	Tempo Intervals	2 x 3 miles with 3 minutes rest	PL (pg. 80)	SR (pg. 33)
	Sa	Rest or Cross-Training	Rest or 30 minutes cross-training		
	Su	Long	10-mile run	PD (pg. 66)	SS (pg. 43) or AS (pg. 49)
WEEK 12	**M**	Easy	4 miles easy	CR (pg. 79)	PR (pg. 21)
	Tu	Long Tempo	3 miles tempo	LB (pg. 79)	SS (pg. 43) or AS (pg. 49)
	W	Rest or Cross-Training	Rest or 30 minutes cross-training		
	Th	Easy	3 miles easy	QR (pg. 66)	PR (pg. 21)
	F	Rest Day	Rest		
	Sa	Easy	2 miles easy		AS (pg. 49)
	Su	Race Day	Race Day		

RESOURCES

These resources have influenced my running philosophy and can be especially helpful to beginners and runners who want to learn more about the subjects covered in this book and beyond.

Books

Anatomy for Runners: Unlocking Your Athletic Potential for Health, Speed, and Injury Prevention by Jay Dicharry

Daniels' Running Formula by Jack Daniels

80/20 Running: Run Stronger and Race Faster by Training Slower by Matt Fitzgerald

Endure: Mind, Body, and the Curiously Elastic Limits of Human Performance by Alex Hutchinson

Explosive Running: Using the Science of Kinesiology to Improve Your Performance by Michael Yessis

Lore of Running by Tim Noakes

Relentless Forward Progress: A Guide to Running Ultramarathons by Bryon Powell

Run Faster from 5k to the Marathon: How to Be Your Own Best Coach by Brad Hudson and Matt Fitzgerald

Running to the Top by Arthur Lydiard

The Runner's Body: How the Latest Exercise Science Can Help You Run Stronger, Longer, and Faster by Ross Tucker and Jonathan Dugas (*Runner's World* book)

Your Best Stride: How to Optimize Your Natural Running Form to Run Easier, Farther, and Faster—With Fewer Injuries by Jonathan Beverly (*Runner's World* book)

Websites

Runners Connect (for video demonstration of drills): https://www.runnersconnect.net/drills/

Run Guides (for fun runs): http://www.runguides.com

Runner's World: https://www.runnersworld.com/

The Science of Running: https://www.scienceofrunning.com/

REFERENCES

Behm, D. G., and A. Chaouachi. "A Review of the Acute Effects of Static and Dynamic Stretching on Performance." *European Journal of Applied Physiology* 111, no. 11 (2011): 2633–51.

Bolívar, Y. A., P. V. Munuera Martínez, and J. P. Padillo. "Relationship between Tightness of the Posterior Muscles of the Lower Limb and Plantar Fasciitis." *Foot & Ankle International* 34, no. 1 (2013): 42–48.

Cichanowski, H. R., J. S. Schmitt, R. J. Johnson, and P. E. Niemuth. "Hip Strength in Collegiate Female Athletes with Patellofemoral Pain." *Medicine & Science in Sports & Exercise* 39, no. 8 (2007): 1227–32.

Derrick, T. R. "The Effects of Knee Contact Angle on Impact Forces and Accelerations." *Medicine & Science in Sports & Exercise* 36, no. 5 (2004): 832–37.

Dudley, G. A., W. M. Abraham, and R. L. Terjung. "Influence of Exercise Intensity and Duration on Biochemical Adaptations in Skeletal Muscle." *Journal of Applied Physiology* 53, no. 4 (1982): 844–50.

Fairclough, J., K. Hayashi, H. Toumi, K. Lyons, G. Bydder, N. Phillips, T. M. Best, and M. Benjamin. "Is Iliotibial Band Syndrome Really a Friction Syndrome?" *Journal of Science and Medicine in Sport* 10, no. 2 (2007): 74–76.

Ferruati, A., M. Bergermann, and J. Fernandez-Fernandez. "Effects of a Concurrent Strength and Endurance Training on Running Performance and Running Economy in Recreational Marathon Runners." *Journal of Strength and Conditioning Research* 24, no. 10 (2010): 2770–78.

Franz, Jason, Kate W. Paylo, Jay Dicharry, Patrick O. Riley, and D. Casey Kerrigan. "Changes in the Coordination of Hip and Pelvis Kinematics with Mode of Locomotion." *Gait & Posture* 29, no. 3 (2009): 494–98.

Fredericson, M., C. L. Cookingham, A. M. Chaudhari, B. C. Dowdell, N. Oestreicher, and S. A. Sahrmann. "Hip Abductor Weakness in Distance Runners with Iliotibial Band Syndrome." *Clinical Journal of Sports Medicine* 10 (2000): 169–75.

Gosztyla A. E., D. G. Edwards, T. J. Quinn, and R. W. Kenefick. "The Impact of Different Pacing Strategies on Five-Kilometer Running Time Trial Performance." *Journal of Strength and Conditioning Research* 20, no. 4 (November 2006): 882–86.

Hasegawa, H., T. Yamauchi, and W. J. Kraemer. "Foot Strike Patterns of Runners at the 15-km Point during an Elite-Level Half Marathon." *Journal of Strength and Conditioning Research* 21 (2007): 888–93.

Heiderscheit B. C., E. S. Chumanov, M. P. Michalski, C. M. Wille, and M. B. Ryan. "Effects of Step Rate Manipulation on Joint Mechanics during Running." *Medicine & Science in Sports & Exercise* 43, no. 2 (February 2011): 296–302.

Ireland, M. L., J. D. Willson, B. T. Ballantyne, and I. S. Davis. "Hip Strength in Females with and without Patellofemoral Pain." *Journal of Orthopaedic & Sports Physical Therapy* 33 (2003): 671–76.

Johnston, R. E., T. J. Quinn, R. Kertzer, and N. B. Vroman. "Strength Training in Female Distance Runners: Impact on Running Economy." *Journal of Strength and Conditioning Research* 11, no. 4 (1997): 224–29.

Jung, A. P. "The Impact of Resistance Training on Distance Running Performance." *Sports Medicine* 33, no. 7 (2003): 539–52.

Kerr, B. A., L. Beauchamp, V. Fisher, and R. Neil. "Footstrike Patterns in Distance Running." In *Biomechanical Aspects of Sport Shoes and Playing Surfaces*, edited by B. M. Nigg, 135–42. Calgary: University Press of Calgary, 1983.

Labovitz, J. M., and J. Yu. "The Role of Hamstring Tightness in Plantar Fasciitis." *Foot & Ankle Specialist* 4, no. 3 (2011): 141–44.

Larson, P., E. Higgins, J. Kaminski, T. Decker, J. Preble, D. Lyons, K. McIntyre, and A. Normile. "Foot Strike Patterns of Recreational and Sub-elite Runners in a Long-Distance Road Race." *Journal of Sports Sciences* 29 (2011): 1665–73.

Larson, Peter. "Gait Variability among Elite Runners at the 2011 Boston Marathon." *Runblogger*. May 3, 2011. https://runblogger.com/2011/05/gait-variability-among-elite-runners-at.html.

Myer, G. D., K. R. Ford, J. P. Palumbo, and T. E. Hewett. "Neuromuscular Training Improves Performance and Lower-Extremity Biomechanics in Female Athletes." *Journal of Strength and Conditioning Research* 19, no. 1 (2005): 51–60.

Niemuth, P. E., R. J. Johnson, M. J. Myers, and T. J. Thieman. "Hip Muscle Weakness and Overuse Injuries in Recreational Runners." *Clinical Journal of Sports Medicine* 15 (2005): 14–21.

Paavolainen, L., K. Häkkinen, I. Hämäläinen, A. Nummela, and H. Rusko. "Explosive-Strength Training Improves 5-km Running Time by Improving Running Economy and Muscle Power." *Journal of Applied Physiology* 86 (1999): 1527–33.

Pereles, D., A. Roth, and D. J. Thompson. "A Large, Randomized, Prospective Study of the Impact of a Pre-run Stretch on the Risk of Injury in Teenage and Older Runners." USA Track and Field, 2010. http://www.usatf.org/stretchstudy/StretchStudyReport.pdf.

Pope, R. "A Randomized Trial of Preexercise Stretching for Prevention of Lower-Limb Injury." *Medicine & Science in Sports & Exercise* 32, no. 2 (2000): 271–77.

Sato, K., and M. Mokha. "Does Core Strength Training Influence Running Kinetics, Lower-Extremity Stability, and 5000-m Performance in Runners?" *Journal of Strength and Conditioning Research* 23, no. 1 (2009):133–40.

Saunders, P. U., R. D. Telford, D. B. Pyne, E. M. Peltola, R. B. Cunningham, C. J. Gore, and J. A. Hawley. "Short-Term Plyometric Training Improves Running Economy in Highly Trained Middle and Long Distance Runners." *Journal of Strength and Conditioning Research* 20, no. 4 (2006): 947–54.

Selkowitz, D. M., G. J. Beneck, and C. M. Powers. "Which Exercises Target the Gluteal Muscles While Minimizing Activation of the Tensor Fascia Lata? Electromyographic Assessment Using Fine-Wire Electrodes." *Journal of Orthopaedic & Sports Physical Therapy* 43, no. 2 (2013): 54–64.

Støren, Ø., J. A. N. Helgerud, E. M. Støa, and J. A. N. Hoff. "Maximal Strength Training Improves Running Economy in Distance Runners." *Medicine & Science in Sports & Exercise* 40, no. 6 (2008): 1087–92.

Turner, A. M., M. Owings, and J. A. Schwane. "Improvement in Running Economy After 6 Weeks of Plyometric Training." *Journal of Strength and Conditioning Research* 17, no. 1 (2003): 60–67.

van Gent, R. N., D. Siem, M. van Middelkoop, A. G. van Os, S. M. A. Bierma-Zeinstra, and B. W. Koes. "Incidence and Determinants of Lower Extremity Running Injuries in Long Distance Runners: A Systematic Review." *British Journal of Sports Medicine* 41, no. 8 (2007): 469–80.

Verrall, G. M., J. P. Slavotinek, and P G Barnes. "The Effect of Sports Specific Training on Reducing the Incidence of Hamstring Injuries in Professional Australian Rules Football Players." *British Journal of Sports Medicine* 39, no. 6 (May 23, 2005): 363–68. https://doi.org/10.1136/bjsm.2005.018697.

Witvrouw, E., J. Bellemans, R. Lysens, L. Danneels, and D. Cambier. "Intrinsic Risk Factors for the Development of Patellar Tendinitis in an Athletic Population: A Two-Year Prospective Study." *American Journal of Sports Medicine* 29, no. 2 (2001): 190–95.

Witvrouw, E., R. Lysens, J. Bellemans, D. Cambier, and G. Vanderstraeten. "Intrinsic Risk Factors for the Development of Anterior Knee Pain in an Athletic Population: A Two-Year Prospective Study." *American Journal of Sports Medicine* 28 (2000): 480–89.

INDEX

ACKNOWLEDGMENTS

This book could not have been written without the support of all the coaches I've had along the way. I appreciate you tolerating my inquisitiveness and fostering my passion for running. I also want to thank my family for their love, support, and patience throughout this process.